History of Toxicology and Environmental Health

History of Toxicology and Environmental Health

Toxicology in Antiquity, Volume I

Philip Wexler

AMSTERDAM • BOSTON • HEIDELBERG • LONDON
NEW YORK • OXFORD • PARIS • SAN DIEGO
SAN FRANCISCO • SINGAPORE • SYDNEY • TOKYO
Academic Press is an imprint of Elsevier

Academic Press is an imprint of Elsevier
225 Wyman Street, Waltham, MA 02451, USA
525 B Street, Suite 1800, San Diego, CA 92101, USA
The Boulevard, Langford Lane, Kidlington, Oxford, OX5 1GB, UK
32 Jamestown Road, London NW1 7BY, UK
Radarweg 29, 1043 NX Amsterdam, The Netherlands

British Library Cataloguing in Publication Data
A catalogue record for this book is available from the British Library

Library of Congress Cataloging-in-Publication Data
A catalog record for this book is available from the Library of Congress

ISBN: 978-0-12-800045-8

For information on all Academic Press publications
visit our website at **store.elsevier.com**

This book has been manufactured using Print On Demand technology. Each copy is produced to order and is limited to black ink. The online version of this book will show color figures where appropriate.

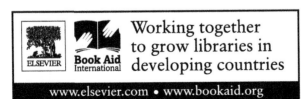

Working together
to grow libraries in
developing countries

www.elsevier.com • www.bookaid.org

TOXICOLOGY IN ANTIQUITY

Dedication—For Nancy, Yetty, Will, Jake, and Lola

With appreciation to the Toxicology History Association and the scholarly contributors to this series

Many thanks, as well, to Elsevier, in particular Molly McLaughlin, for expertly navigating us through the publication terrain.

CONTENTS

LIST OF CONTRIBUTORS

Adrienne Mayor
Research scholar, Classics Department and History and Philosophy of Science and Technology Program, Stanford University, Stanford, California, USA

Alain Touwaide
Institute for the Preservation of Medical Traditions and Smithsonian Institution, Washington, D.C., USA

Benny Pfanz, BSc
Faculty of Geosciences, Ruhr-University, Bochum, Germany

W. Benson Harer
Former Clinical Professor of Obstetrics and Gynecology, Western University of Health Sciences, Pomona, California, USA; Former Adjunct Professor of Egyptian Art at California State University, San Bernardino, California, USA

Francesco D'Andria
Prof. Dr., University of Salento, Italy; Department of Cultural Heritage, Director of the Italian Archaeological Mission in Hierapolis of Phrygia, Turkey

Francois Retief
Honorary Research Fellow, Department of Greek, Latin and Classical Studies, University of the Free State, Bloemfontein, South Africa

Galip Yüce
Professor, Hacettepe University, Faculty of Engineering, Department of Geological Engineering, Hydrogeology Division, Beytepe, Ankara, Turkey

George Androutsos
Professor and Chairman, History of Medicine Department, Medical School, National and Kapodistrian, University of Athens, Athens, Greece

George Papatheodorou
Prof. Dr., Laboratory of Marine Geology and Physical Oceanography, University of Patras, Patras, Greece

Gonzalo M. Sanchez
(Retired from) Avera Medical Group, Pierre, South Dakota, USA

Gregory Tsoucalas
Faculty of Medicine, History of Medicine, University of Thessaly, Larissa, Greece

Hardy Pfanz
Prof. Dr., Chair of Applied Botany, Director of Botanic Gardens, University of Duisburg-Essen, Campus Essen, Essen, Germany

Jelle Zeilinga de Boer
Harold T. Stearns Professor of Earth Science, Emeritus, Wesleyan University, Middletown, Connecticut, USA

Louise Cilliers
Honorary Research Fellow, Department of Greek, Latin and Classical Studies, University of the Free State, Bloemfontein, South Africa

Marianna Karamanou
Scientific Collaborator, History of Medicine Department, Medical School, National and Kapodistrian University of Athens, Athens, Greece

Markos Sgantzos
Faculty of Medicine, History of Medicine, University of Thessaly, Larissa, Greece

Okan Arihan
Faculty of Medicine, Department of Physiology, Yuzuncu Yil University, Turkey

Seda Karaoz Arihan
Faculty of Letters, Department of Anthropology, Yuzuncu Yil University, Turkey

Walter D'Alessandro
Dr., Instituto di Geofisica e Vulcanologia, Sezione di Palermo, Palermo, Italy

Yiannis Manetas
Prof. Dr., Laboratory of Plant Physiology, Department of Biology, University of Patras, Patras, Greece

Henry Ford was famously contemptuous of history. He is on record as saying, "History is more or less bunk. It's tradition. We don't want tradition. We want to live in the present and the only history that is worth a tinker's damn is the history we make today." Personally I prefer George Santayana's view: "...[W]hen experience is not retained, as among savages, infancy is perpetual. Those who cannot remember the past are condemned to repeat it." But how relevant is historical toxicology? What can we modern toxicologists (and our regulatory authorities) learn from the past? One important lesson is that toxicity can affect people anywhere, in any society, at any level, and for many years, without anyone being aware of it. Toxic effects on the brain may be responsible for misjudgments by political leaders that can have disastrous consequences. Toxicity may have caused the fall of empires. Jerome Nriagu [1] has argued in his 1983 book that "lead poisoning contributed to the decline of the Roman empire." Louise Cilliers, in Volume 1 of this series, though, disagrees with Nriagu's conclusion. Thus, we must consider further the Roman emperors' possible exposure to other toxicants described by Cilliers and Retief in an earlier article [2]. Maybe excessive wine consumption was enough to explain the emperors' self-destructive behavior. Maybe the effects of ethanol were supplemented by the effects of opium, widely used in ancient Rome as a soporific and an analgesic as well as an aid to digestion [2]. There is clearly still much scope for further research in this area.

Another empire that may have suffered the consequences of toxicity at the highest level is that of China. It seems possible that the latter days and decisions of the Chinese Emperor Qin Shi Huang may have been adversely affected by exposure to mercury. According to the historian Sima Qian, this emperor was buried in a mausoleum with 100 rivers of flowing mercury in addition to his now famous "terra cotta army." Reportedly, Qin Shi Huang died as a result of ingesting mercury pills, prescribed by his alchemists and court physicians in order to make him immortal [3]. It is not unreasonable to suppose, based on his interest in flowing mercury, which probably was to be found in his palace as well as his mausoleum, that some time before his death he was already suffering from mercury poisoning and that his mental function and judgment were impaired as a consequence. It is also likely that his son, the succeeding Emperor Qin Er Shi, had suffered exposure to mercury in his father's palace and that this led to his ill-judged decisions—for example, his command to lacquer the city walls [4]. In any event, his incompetence led to revolt, he was forced to commit suicide, and the Qin Dynasty and Empire came to an end, with the Qin capital being destroyed by rebels [4].

With these thoughts in mind, all toxicologists and all those concerned with human health, the environment, and the possible influence of toxic human environments on our political leaders must welcome the insights from history that this first volume and succeeding volumes in this new series of publications will bring. Frequently, I hear toxicologists remark that they might have reached better conclusions in the past "with the benefit of hindsight." Now that this series will give us the all the benefit of hindsight, no doubt "better conclusions" will follow.

John Duffus
The Edinburgh Centre for Toxicology

REFERENCES

[1] Nriagu JO. Saturnine gout among Roman aristocrats. Did lead poisoning contribute to the fall of the Empire? N Engl J Med 1983;308(11):660−3.

[2] Cilliers L, Retief FP. Poisons, poisoning and the drug trade in ancient Rome. Akroterion 2000;45:88−100.

[3] Wright DC. The history of China. Greenwood Publishing Group, Westport, CT; 2001; 264 pp. ISBN 0-313-30940-X.

[4] Hardy G, Kinney AB. The establishment of the Han Empire and Imperial China. Greenwood Publishing Group, Westport, CT; 2005; 170 pp. ISBN 031332588X.

In the realm of communicating any science, history, though critical to its progress, is typically a neglected backwater. This is unfortunate, as it can easily be the most fascinating, revealing, and accessible aspect of a subject which might otherwise hold appeal for only a highly specialized technical audience. Toxicology, the science concerned with the potentially hazardous effects of chemical, biological, and certain physical agents, has yet to be the subject of a full-scale historical treatment. Overlapping with many other sciences, it both draws from and contributes to them. Chemistry, biology, and pharmacology all intersect with toxicology. While there have been chapters devoted to history in toxicology textbooks, and journal articles have filled in bits and pieces of the historical record, this new monographic series aims to further remedy the gap by offering an extensive and systematic look at the subject from antiquity to the present.

Since ancient times, men and women have sought security of all kinds. This includes identifying and making use of beneficial substances while avoiding the harmful ones, or mitigating harm already caused. Thus, food and other natural products, independently or in combination, which promoted well-being or were found to have drug-like properties and effected cures, were readily consumed, applied, or otherwise self-administered or made available to friends and family. On the other hand, agents found to cause injury or damage—what we might call *poisons* today—were personally avoided although sometimes employed to wreak havoc upon one's enemies.

While natural substances are still of toxicological concern, synthetic and industrial chemicals now predominate as the emphasis of research. Through the years, the instinctive human need to seek safety and avoid hazard has served as an unchanging foundation for toxicology, and will be explored from many angles in this series. Although largely examining the scientific underpinnings of the field, chapters will also delve into the fascinating history of toxicology and poisons in mythology, arts, society, and culture more broadly. It is a subject that has captured our collective consciousness.

The series is intentionally broad, thus the title *History of Toxicology and Environmental Health*. Clinical and research toxicology, environmental and occupational health, risk assessment, and epidemiology, to name but a few examples, are all fair game subjects for inclusion. Volumes 1 and 2 focus on toxicology in antiquity, taken roughly to be the period up to the fall of the Roman empire and stopping short of the Middle Ages, with which period future volumes will continue. These opening volumes will explore toxicology from the perspective of some of the great civilizations of the past, including Egypt, Greece, Rome, Mesoamerica, and China. Particular substances, such as harmful botanicals, lead, cosmetics, kohl, and hallucinogens, serve as the focus of other chapters. The role of certain individuals as either victims or practitioners of toxicity (e.g., Cleopatra, Mithridates, Alexander the Great, Socrates, and Shen Nung) serves as another thrust of these volumes.

History proves that no science is static. As Nikola Tesla said, "The history of science shows that theories are perishable. With every new truth that is revealed we get a better understanding of Nature and our conceptions and views are modified."

Great research derives from great researchers who do not, and cannot, operate in a vacuum, but rely on the findings of their scientific forebears. To quote Sir Isaac Newton, "If I have seen further it is by standing on the shoulders of giants."

Welcome to this toxicological journey through time. You will surely see further and deeper and more insightfully by wafting through the waters of toxicology's history.

Phil Wexler

CHAPTER *1*

Toxicology in Ancient Egypt

Gonzalo M. Sanchez and W. Benson Harer

1.1 INTRODUCTION

The ancient Egyptians were astute observers of natural phenomena. The ability to incorporate these observations into their beliefs about religion, politics, and magic was a major factor in the survival of their culture for so many centuries. *Maat* was their term for the proper order of things in the world.

Poisonous snakes and insects posed a special challenge to incorporate into a proper order of the universe. The Egyptians' solution to incorporating them into their belief system was to be able to control them by magic. The scorpion became the goddess Selket, one of the guardians of the king's sarcophagus. At least 10 gods and goddesses who could be protective were portrayed with serpent heads. The king, for example, converted the cobra to his protector. The horned viper was the hieroglyph word for the masculine designation as well as for the letter "f." When the horned viper depiction in a glyph was needed in an inscription in a tomb, there was a perceived risk that it could come to life to bite the owner so it might be portrayed with the head severed from the body to be safe. Magic, or "ritual power," was produced to protect the deceased from the most dangerous entity of all, the serpent Apophis, who threatened to block the king's passage through the dangerous night to rebirth in the afterlife.

1.2 SNAKES AS DESCRIBED IN THE BROOKLYN PAPYRUS

The study of venomous snakebite, its chemistry, its mode of action, and the biology of the venom-producing organism are considered part of the science currently known as toxinology. The Brooklyn Museum Papyri, ca. 525−600 BCE, consist of two sections, 47,218.48 and 47,218.85, which describe individual snakes and treatment for snakebites, respectively [1]. These papyri, translated by Sauneron [2], are our major source of information on snakebites in ancient Egypt.

History of Toxicology and Environmental Health. DOI: http://dx.doi.org/10.1016/B978-0-12-800045-8.00001-0

The Brooklyn Papyri originally contained 100 paragraphs; §1–13 are missing, but presumably contained material similar to that found in §14–38. A summary of the information included therein is as follows:

Paragraphs 14–37:

1. Snake identification by name; physical characteristics of size, color, shape of the head, neck; bite marks; behavior; reptation (i.e., the manner in which it crawls); aggressiveness; and the snake's state of alertness (some text is missing).
2. Effects of the bite, local symptoms (swelling, bleeding, pain, necrosis, and discoloration), and systemic symptoms (fever, vomiting, fainting, loss of strength, loss of consciousness, tetanization, possible seizures, and coma).
3. Prognoses and recommendation of initial treatment.

Paragraph 38: Description is of a chameleon, not a snake.

Paragraphs 39–100 include treatments for the snakebites described.

1.2.1 Snake Identification

Identification of snakes from ancient Egyptian descriptions in sections 47, 218, and 48 of the Brooklyn Papyri are not established with certainty. In paragraphs 13–37, Sauneron [2, p. 164, 165] labels his identification of 18 of them as "probable" and his identification of four of them as "possible." Likewise, Nunn and Warrell identify 13 of these and label those as tentative identifications [3, p. 183–6]. An example of certainty in snake identification is shown in parallel texts §28 [2, p. 25] and the contemporary description of *Cerastes cerastes* [4, p. 121–3] (Figure 1.1).

The snake identification in the Brooklyn Papyri has raised an interesting issue with the snake in §15, Apophis, as this snake features most prominently in the mythology of ancient Egypt as the personification of evil. Apophis is represented in the various royal tombs and in the Book of the Dead, with consistent morphological characteristics: a large snake with a small head, large eye, and round pupil. The body is dark on top with a distinct light underbelly. Apophis in the Brooklyn Papyri [2, p. 9] is described as a large snake, reddish brown in color, with a light underbelly, having four fangs and a lethal bite. Regarding the identification of the snake in §15, John Nunn [3, p. 185] remarks, "A positive identification would be valuable, but no Egyptian snake

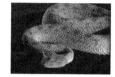

fy ḥr dbwy

(Viper with Horns)

Sahara Horned Viper

Cerastes cerastes

Regarding a *Viper with horns,* its color is similar to that of a quail; it has two horns [on] its forehead; its head is broad, his neck is narrow, [his] tail is thick.
(If) the orifice of his bite is broad, the face of the injured swells; (if) its bite is small, one who was bitten becomes inert, but [...] (?)...]. Fever for nine days, (but) he will survive. It is a manifestation of Horus. Its venom is [out] attracted by making him vomit profusely, and exorcizing[...].

A short stout viper, the head is broad, flat and triangular, the eye is prominent on the side of the head, and has a vertical pupil in bright light. The neck is thin. The body is broad and flattened, tail short. There is a long horn above each eye, this horn consists of a single scale. Ground color, yellowish, biscuit colored with brown blotches along its back.
Bites involve swelling and hemorrhage, and necrosis at bite site. Nausea and vomiting occur. Hematuria. Fatalities are infrequent.

Serge Sauneron. Papyrus du Musee de Brooklyn No 47.218.48 + 85 Premiere Parte. Paragraph 28, p.25.1989 Hieratic text translation.

Partial text from S. Spawls and B. Branch "The Dangerous Snakes of Africa," 1995

Figure 1.1 Sahara Horned Viper. Comparative text from the Brooklyn Papyri with a contemporary source. Photo by Gonzalo M. Sanchez, author.

fits the description. The largest and most rapidly fatal snake is the Egyptian cobra." The two large dangerous snakes currently in Egypt are the Egyptian Cobra and the Desert Black Snake [4, p. 69, 70, 87; 5, p. 155, 156, 188]. Although we agree with Nunn that "no Egyptian snake fits the description" of the snake in Brooklyn Papyri §15, it is possible that such a snake can be found in Sudan. The desertification shift occurring in Southern Egypt in the last five millennia resulted in its flora and fauna retreating to Sudan [2, p. 146; 6, p. 45]. Four large venomous snakes found today in Sudan are the Black Mamba, Puff Adder, Black Spitting Cobra, and Boomslang [5, p. 165, 194, 198, 203]. While no longer found in Egypt, the Puff Adder can be easily identified as the snake in §33 [2, p. 29]. Of these four snakes, only the Boomslang (*Dyspholidus typhus* in the Colubridae family) has those physical characteristics that could correspond to the snake in §15, Apophis (Figure 1.2).

1.2.2 Symptoms of Snakebite
The Brooklyn Papyri and other Egyptian texts demonstrate that the ancient Egyptians recognized the different symptoms and signs of

Papyrus du Musée de Brooklyn No 47.218.48 + 85 Premiere Partie § 15

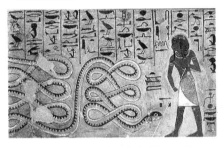

[Quant] au grand serpent d'Âpopi, il est rouge en totalité*; son ventre est blanc**; il y a quatre crocs dans sa bouche. S'il mord quelqu'un, celui-ci meurt aussiôt.

* a chromatic gamma near red, brown, bronze, reddish-brown
** white, whitish, cream.

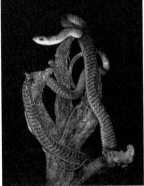

Dispholidus typhus

Boomslang

Rear-fanged snake Highly variable in coloration, from green to dark brown or black above with a pale belly. Eyes very large, round pupils. Most dangerous of Africa's Colubridae family. Its venom is hemotoxic.

The god Atum spearing Apophis – Tomb of Ramses I, Luxor, Egypt.

Photo courtesy:
Terry Philip, Curator,
Black Hills Reptile Gardens
Rapid City S.D.

Figure 1.2 Brooklyn Papyri serpent Apophis, comparison with Boomslang. Reproduction of the god Atum spearing the serpent Apophis from the tomb of pharaoh Ramses I in Luxor, Egypt is from public domain file: Apep 1 jpg, from Wikipedia Commons. The composite hieroglyph text and legends done by Gonzalo M. Sanchez, author. The Boomslang snake photo in this regarding Apophis is used with permission from his owner Travis Phillip. Permission filed.

serious snake envenomation according to their source: vipers or cobras and related snakes (elapids). An example is found in the legend of the god Ra suffering the effects of viper envenomation after having been struck by a snake [7, p. 324, 325].

Today, we understand that these clinical effects are due to the main toxic components of the specific venoms in the various snake families, predominantly hemotoxins in vipers and neurotoxins in elapids.

Viper venom causes tissue damage at the bite site and in its proximity, with changes in red blood cells, defects in coagulation, and damage to blood vessels and often to the heart, kidneys, and lungs.

Neurotoxic venoms of elapid snakes (i.e., cobras) cause lesser local tissue damage, but rapid alterations to the nervous system, secondary cardiac and respiratory failure, and death.

1.2.3 Prognosis

- "He will die immediately": (§15, 16, 17) [2, p. 9–12]. "Death hastens very quickly" (§19) [2, p. 14].
- "He will live": (§22, 25, 26, 28) [2, p. 16, 21, 22, 25]. "One does not die because of it": (§21, 32, 33, 37) [2, p. 15, 28, 29, 33, 34].
- "One can save him" (uncertain): (§14, 18, 20, 24, 27, 29, 30, 31, 33, 34) [2, p. 7, 13, 14, 19, 20, 23, 26, 27, 29–31].

The prognosis of the number of days the patient could survive is sometimes related to whether or not he vomited and whether magic could be administered [2, p. 180, 181].

1.2.4 Treatment [2, p. 180–213]

Some treatments were for any snakebite and some were snake specific.

Bites by the lethal snakes §15, 16, 17, 19 received no treatment [2, p. 9–12, 14]. The bite by snake §33 received treatment, except when the patient had developed signs of what today we understand to be cranial nerve dysfunction [2, p. 29, 30]. Magic is considered useful in §17 [2, p. 186–8].

Therapeutic measures, whether local or systemic, were primarily symptomatic. In viper bites, local edema, necrosis, weakness, sweating, tremors, bleeding, thirst, fever, and pain were treated. In elapid bites, treatment was intended for paralysis, dyspnea, heart failure, aphasia, and seizures.

For local wounds, the bite site was treated with medications kept in place by bandages, with fumigations, and sometimes with incisions or debridement over which medications were applied (§31, 32) [2, p. 27–9]. No tourniquets were used.

Discussion of the extensive pharmacopeia included in the Brooklyn Papyri is beyond the scope of this chapter. Because of the extensive use of Allii Cepae, the onion, it will be addressed here. Onion/water preparations were applied to the bite from the snake identified as Sekhtef §46 in the treatment section only [2, p. 41]. This snake is not listed in the extant section on snake identification due to the loss of paragraphs 1–13. Onion was also used in coating and fumigating the bite of the Black Spitting Cobra §47g, 82b; [2, p. 42, 48] in compresses for *Echis coloratus* §48c bite; [2, p. 42] in bites of "any venomous snake" §92, 95b; [2, p. 50] and particularly with copper fillings to the bite of the Persian viper §51c [2, p. 43].

Possible effects of the topical use of Allii Cepae in snakebite include the following:

a. Phospholipase A2
   Snake venom phospholipase A2 (PLA2) toxins are present in almost all venomous species. Having different tissue targets, these toxins, we know today, can be myotoxic and/or neurotoxic [8, p. 2897−912] and can lyse the phospholipid membranes of red blood cells [9, p. 60−73]. The release of arachidonic acid metabolites produces inflammation [10, p. 947−62]. The topical application of an aqueous extract of *Bulbus Allii Cepae* (10% in a gel preparation) has been found to inhibit mouse ear edema induced by arachidonic acid. The flavonoids quercetin and kaempferol in onions inhibit phospholipase A2, or PLA(2), cyclooxygenase, protein kinase, and the release of histamine from leukocytes [11, p. 10].

b. Paralyzing the lymphatic pump
   Large toxin molecules from elapid snake venoms need first to be absorbed and transported into lymphatic vessels before entering the bloodstream [12, p. 183−5]. The current use of pressure immobilization in elapid snakebites is done for the purpose of impeding lymphatic transport without compromising arterial blood flow, thereby delaying toxins entering the circulation [13, p. 809−11]. Slowing of the lymphatic pump up to 400% by topical use of ointment containing glyceryl trinatrate, which releases nitric oxide, has been demonstrated by Australian investigators led by Dirk van Helden [13]. Thus, the release of nitric oxide from *S*-nitrosoglutathione contained in extracts of aqueous garlic, onion, and leek [14, p. 396−402] could explain some benefit from the use of topical applications of aqueous onion in elapid snakebites by the ancient Egyptians. The nitric oxide effect on the lymphatic pump would have been at least temporarily beneficial.

   Believing that onion would kill the venom of any snake (§42) [2, p. 186] and that vomiting would get rid of the poison, the ancient Egyptians often used emetics and onions in the systemic treatment of snakebite. Recent research has demonstrated the plausibility of onion as a therapeutic agent. In ancient Egypt, onion mixed with beer (and other substances), for example, was ingested and then vomited after a specified period of time [2, p. 56, 57, 66, 69, 72, 74, 76, 83, 84]. Texeira 10 found that oral administration of an ethanol extract of onions to guinea pigs inhibited smooth muscle contractions in the trachea and also inhibited histamine-, serotonin-, and acetylcholine-induced contractions in the ileum.

1.3 SCORPIONS
1.3.1 The Berlin Papyrus
The Berlin Medical Papyrus [15, p. 278] (ca. 1200 BCE) is a general medical document that parallels the medical content of the Ebers Medical papyrus. Its paragraph §78 lists unknown ingredients used for fumigation treatment of a scorpion "bite." Other treatments given for scorpion sting in the Egyptian literature are magic incantations, like the "Spell for conjuring a cat," [16, p. 15] which involved repelling the poison by magic, along with the use of fabric and incisions to remove the venom.

1.4 TETANUS

Tetanus infection developing as a complication of an open wound is addressed in the Edwin Smith Papyrus Case No. 7 [17, p. 71−85]. This document (ca. 1650−1550), currently housed at the New York Academy of Medicine, is the second major text related to ancient Egyptian medicine. It is a copy of the older original (date range 2200−2000 BCE) which has not been found. The Edwin Smith Papyrus, the first comprehensive trauma treatise in the history of medicine, presents a pragmatic approach to the classification and management of head, neck, and upper body injuries and is the source of numerous anatomical and functional concepts of the nervous system. In Case No. 7, the ancient Egyptians appear to extend the concept of illness originating from penetration of the body (by unknown entity) through an open cranial wound, resulting in the development of symptoms of tetanus "because of that wound...." They understood the effects of tetanus and the futility of treatment, even though the nature of this toxin would not be known for millennia.

1.5 PLANT AND MINERAL TOXINS

The ancient Egyptians did not embrace poisoning as a means of execution or assassination as was later done by the Greeks and Romans. A possible exception is the much-discussed murder of Ramses III in a conspiracy hatched in his harem [18]. The trial of the perpetrators was documented and indicates that he survived for 2 weeks after the attempt by unspecified means involving magic. This suggests the use of a slow-acting poison such as ricin, found in the seed of the castor plant. The Egyptians were probably aware of the danger of the castor bean since they understood the use of castor oil as medicine. A magical incantation was considered essential to activate ingredients.

Dosage determines the ranges of therapeutic action and toxicity of drugs. The Ebers Papyrus [19], dated to 1536 BCE (the 9th year of the reign of Amenophis I), is the most voluminous papyrus document known. It is a medical text that provides over 800 recipes to treat almost any symptom imaginable. All the components were dispensed by volume rather than weight, and treatments could be administered by mouth, anal, or vaginal suppository, by lotion or ointment applied to the skin, or even by fumigation as smoke. A critical element, however, is that they be accompanied by an incantation to assure their efficacy. Therapeutic or toxic effects were dependent on the degree of absorption into the patient's body. Experience would have permitted them to avoid toxic levels of drugs such as wormwood, hyoscyamine, and mandrake, but no actual references to toxicity were made.

Alcohol is well understood for its dose-related toxicity. The Egyptians consumed it in both beer and wine. Indeed, beer was a staple of their diet. Their writings berate overindulgence and they were aware that alcohol could be habit forming. Wine was the drink of the elite. Both were used as vehicles for many prescriptions. Their beer probably contained about 5% alcohol and their wine 10−14%. With those concentrations, they probably didn't drink sufficient amounts to raise the blood alcohol to a lethal level. We know of no account of death from alcohol poisoning.

It appears that they understood that some of their therapeutic alkaloids were soluble only in alcohol, and used beer or wine as vehicles for their delivery. A papyrus in Leiden gives us the original recipe for a "Mickey Finn," a potion to put an unsuspecting person to sleep— mandrake and hyoscyamine steeped in wine [20, p. 148−51]. Another example is the Egyptian "lotus," more accurately described as *Nymphea cerulea* and *Nymphea alba*. Both contain narcotic alkaloids [21, p. 49−54]. The latter are concentrated in the flower, but not in the seeds or leaves. The blue lotus figures prominently in Egyptian mythology, with its yellow stamen mimicking the sun in the blue sky of the petals. Four of its active ingredients have been isolated and studied. While the narcotic properties of the lotus are not well recognized by Egyptologists, there is good evidence that it was understood by the ancients. Two prescriptions in the Ebers papyrus use beer and wine in which it has "spent the night" as the vehicles to carry it. The true Nelumbo lotus, which contains 14 powerful narcotic alkaloids, did not enter Egypt until the Persian conquest in 525 BCE.

In 1934, Dawson [22, p. 185−8] proposed that the word *Shemshemet* could be cannabis. Since then it has figured prominently in literature, but there is absolutely no archeological evidence of cannabis being present in ancient Egypt, even to make rope. There is no evidence it was used as a drug until after the Arab conquest centuries later.

Galena, or lead sulfide, was the black eye paint used for many ophthalmic problems. It was probably also used with soot and other binders to make mascara. Despite its toxicity, the effects from absorption through the skin would be slow to develop. We have no evidence that this danger was recognized by the Egyptians.

REFERENCES

[1] Leitz C. Die Schlangensprueche in den Pyramidentexten. Orientalia (Nova Series) Roma 1996;65:382.

[2] Sauneron S. Un traité Égyptien d'óphiologie. Papyrus du Brooklyn museum nos 47.218.48 et 85. Le Caire: Institut Français d'Archéologie Orientale; 1989. p. 21, 48, 148, 149, 164, 165.

[3] Nunn JF. Ancient Egyptian medicine. Norman, OK: University of Oklahoma Press; 1996. p. 183−6.

[4] Spawls S, Branch B. The dangerous snakes of Africa. South Africa: Southern Book Publishers Ltd.; 1995. p. 69, 70, 87, 121−3.

[5] Shupe S. Venomous snakes of the world. New York, NY: Skyhorse Publishing; 2013. p. 155, 156, 165, 194, 198, 203.

[6] Houlihan PF. The animal world of the pharaohs. Cairo: The American University in Cairo Press; 1995. p. 45.

[7] Oakes L, Gahlin L. Isis and the sun god's secret name. Ancient Egypt. New York, NY: Anness Publishing, Barnes and Noble; 2006. p. 324, 325.

[8] Montecucco C, Gutierrez GM, Lomonte B. Cellular pathology induced by snake venom phospholipase A2 myotoxins and neurotoxins: common aspects of their mechanisms of action. Cell Mol Life Sci 2008;18:2897−912.

[9] Condrea E, De Vries A, Magner J. Hemolysis by lysing the phospholipid cell membranes of red blood cells. Specialized section on lipids and related subjects. Biochim Biophys Acta 1964;84:60−73.

[10] Texeira CF, Landucci EC, Antunes E, Chacur M, Cury Y. Inflammatory effects of snake venom myotoxic phospholipases A2. Toxicon 2003;42(8):947−62.

[11] WHO. Bulbus Allii Cepae. Monographs on selected medical plants. Geneva: World Health Organization; 1999. p. 10.

[12] Sutherland SK, Coulter AR, Harris RD. Rationalisation of first-aid measures for elapid snakebite. Lancet 1979;1(8109):183−5.

[13] Saul ME, Thomas PA, Dosen PJ, Isbister GK, O'Leary MA, Whyte IM, et al. A pharmacological approach to first aid treatment for snakebite. Nat Med 2011;17(7):809−11.

[14] Grman M, Misak A, Cacanyiova S, Tamascova Z, Bertova A, Ondrias K. The aqueous garlic, onion and leek extracts release nitric oxide from S-nitrosogluthatione and prolong relaxation of aortic rings. Gen Physiol Biophys 2011;(4):396−402.

[15] Westendorf W. Handbuch der Altägyptischen medizin. Leiden/Boston/Koln/Berlin: Brill; 1998. p. 278.

[16] Kousoulis P. Stop, O poison, that I may find your name according to your aspect: a preliminary study on the ambivalent notion of poison and the demonization of the scorpion's sting in ancient Egypt and abroad. J Anc Egypt Interconnections 2011.

[17] Sanchez GM, Meltzer ES. The Edwin Smith Papyrus: updated translation of the trauma treatise and modern medical commentaries. Atlanta, GA: Lockwood Press; 2012. p. 71−85.

[18] Redford S. The harem conspiracy. DeKalb, IL: Northern Illinios University Press; 2002.

[19] Ghalioungi P. The ebers papyrus. Cairo: Academy of Scientific Research and Technology; 1987.

[20] Griffith FL, Thompson H. The Leyden papyrus. New York, NY: Dover Publications; 1974. p. 148−51.

[21] Harer WB. Pharmacological and biological properties of the Egyptian lotus. JARCE 1985;22:49−54.

[22] Dawson WR. Studies in the Egyptian medical texts. JEA 1934;20:185−8.

CHAPTER 2

The Death of Cleopatra: Suicide by Snakebite or Poisoned by Her Enemies?

Gregory Tsoucalas and Markos Sgantzos

2.1 CLEOPATRA'S ANCESTRY AND HISTORICAL BACKGROUND OF THE ERA

Soon after the death of Alexander the Great, his generals ruled a divided empire. One of his favorites, Ptolemy (father of Cleopatra), was assigned to govern Egypt. A supreme dynasty had arisen in this part of the northeast corner of the African continent. Ptolemy had decided to transform the city of Alexandria into the greatest trade, cultural, and religious center of the known world. His plans included the largest harbor of the Mediterranean Sea, majestic palaces, extraordinary public buildings, museums, the wondrous Pharos lighthouse, wide boulevards laid out in a grid, translation centers, libraries, and irrigation and drainage systems. Inside the walls of the famous Library of Alexandria were gathered manuscripts from all over the world to encompass all the known knowledge of the era [1,2].

In this magnificent city, at the prime of its civilization, the great Cleopatra VII (Figure 2.1) was born in 69 BC. At the time of her birth, Rome was perhaps the only city that could be considered a rival to Alexandria. Rome, though, was vastly superior to the Egyptian metropolis, in terms of the magnitude and extent of its military power, which it used to control its vast territories. Meanwhile, Alexandria ruled over Egypt, and over a few of the neighboring coasts and islands. The fruitfulness of this isolated territory, at the magnificent delta of the river Nile, along with its strategic location, made it a perfect target for the Romans. While the idea of a new Roman province was compelling, Egyptian military and strategic power tempered such thoughts. Political events, though, were in their favor and the bountiful prey, Egypt, was lured by Rome and fell into the trap [3].

The Roman government at the time was a republic, and the senate had extended powers. The two most powerful men in the state of Rome

History of Toxicology and Environmental Health. DOI: http://dx.doi.org/10.1016/B978-0-12-800045-8.00002-2

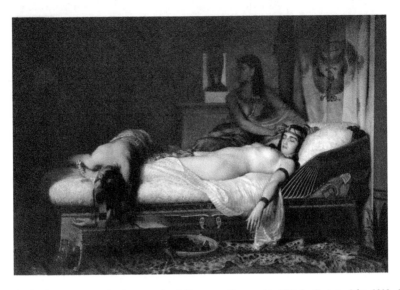

Figure 2.1 On the antique painting in encaustic of Cleopatra, discovered in 1818 by Sartain, John, 1808–1897. Published in 1885 by G. Gebbie & Co. in Philadelphia.

were Pompey and Caesar. Caesar was in the ascendency in Rome when Ptolemy first petitioned him for an alliance between the two great nations of that era, that is, Rome and Egypt. Meanwhile, Pompey was otherwise occupied in Asia Minor, engaged in a war with Mithridates, the powerful monarch of Pontos, who was at that time challenging Rome. Caesar was deep in debt, and much in need of financial resources, not only for relief from existing public embarrassments but also to enable him to accomplish the assorted political schemes which he was entertaining, and to secure his hold on Rome. Negotiations were difficult and delays long, but it was finally agreed that Caesar would exert his influence to secure an alliance between the Roman people and Ptolemy, on the condition that Ptolemy would pay him 6000 talents (ancient Egyptian currency), an enormous amount and, essentially, a bribe. While this served to establish a formal alliance, it also had a serious impact on the Egyptian people. Subsequently, due to an uproar by the citizens over the imposition of heavy taxes, Ptolemy fled to Rome in search of safety. There, a formal alliance was established. The door was then open for Rome to more directly intervene in Egypt [3–5].

During the above turmoil, in 58 BC, with Ptolemy XII absent, his daughter, Berenice, sister of Cleopatra, ascended to the throne. She married the king of Syria, Seleucus, whom she reportedly strangled.

Her second marriage to the prince Archelaus was more successful. Meanwhile, Ptolemy was plotting with the Romans for his return. Although negotiations were difficult, the Romans had decided to permit Pompey to send troops into Egypt. Gabinius, who governed Syria with his second-in-command, Mark Anthony, was a wild and dissolute young man who had lost his family inheritance and embarked on a brief but successful campaign against Egypt. Archelaus was slaughtered in the final ferocious encounter and Berenice was taken prisoner. Cleopatra was only 15 when the unnatural quarrel between her father, Ptolemy, and her sister, Berenice, was working its way toward a dreadful termination. She was a quiet spectator, neither benefitting nor suffering. Ptolemy recaptured the throne. Mark Anthony and the Roman troops remained in Alexandria to help rule a wounded empire [3,6].

In Rome, a civil war between Caesar and Pompey was raging. Cleopatra was the oldest, trusted child, and a princess of great promise, endowed with a sharp intellect and personal charms. In order to retain control over his family legacy, Ptolemy ordered her, before his death, to be married to her brother, Ptolemy XIII, who was only 10 years old at the time. Cleopatra was 18 when she was crowned queen, and rivalry among her ministers inside the royal palace was continuous. Pompey went to Egypt seeking assistance against Caesar but instead was brutally murdered in front of Ptolemy XII, her father, an act that infuriated even Caesar, who subsequently marched against Alexandria [3,6].

Sometime later, Cleopatra and her loyal guardian Apollodorus appeared in front of Caesar to plead for her own agenda in the ensuing power struggle with Ptolemy XII. She forthwith gained Caesar's heart. Caesar made it possible for her to gain Egypt's throne, making Rome appear more an ally than a conqueror. Together they fought against her father, Ptolemy XII, and her minister Pothinus, ultimately securing both their deaths. In 47 BC, Cleopatra gave birth to Caesar's son, Caesarion. Some months later, during a visit with her son to Caesar's palace in an island of the Tiber River, she informed him that she was the undeniable Queen of Egypt, mother of a Roman prince [3,6].

In 44 BC, Caesar was assassinated. Mark Anthony joined with Caesar's adopted son, Octavian, and Lepdius to form the Second Triumvirate. Mark Anthony had already been attracted to Cleopatra and she went on to fully capture his heart. He spent the winter of 41–40 BC, in Egypt, drunk in love with Cleopatra. The couple began to expand Cleopatra's realm through continuous warfare. Anthony soon sent a message to Rome saying that he would abandon his wife (yes, he had a wife back home) to marry his intoxicating concubine, Cleopatra. Rome, specifically Octavian, furiously turned against the couple, declaring yet another war against the Egyptian Empire. After fierce sea battles and violent slaughters on land in the area of western Greece, Cleopatra and Anthony were defeated and retreated back to Egypt. Cleopatra had supported two great Roman leaders and kept Egypt an independent state for some 20 years, but in the end lost everything [3,6].

As Anthony was consumed by his defeat, Cleopatra sent him a message saying that she had died. Eager to save herself, her sons, and the crown from the advancing Octavian, she realized that she could neither kill Anthony nor exile him. But she believed that if he could be induced to kill himself for love of her, she could save herself. And, indeed, Anthony attempted suicide by a self-inflicted sword wound. The injury, though, was not immediately fatal. Discovering that his queen was still alive, he managed to reach her chambers and see her once more before he expired. Octavian had entered Alexandria as a conqueror on August 1, 30 BC. There, at the Palace of the Ptolemies, he found the lifeless body of Mark Anthony and met the notoriously charming queen. Cleopatra, with all her subtlety and political foresight, had already backed two losers, first Caesar and then Anthony, to whose downfall she had notably contributed. Now, at the age of 40, she tried to seduce the new Roman conqueror, Octavian, but he was coldly indifferent toward her advances [3].

Cleopatra understood that she would likely be publicly humiliated as a trophy of Octavian. She remained locked in her mausoleum during her final days, searching for a solution out of this crisis. Two handmaidens and, possibly, a eunuch were with her at the time. Cleopatra ordered a bath and asked for a basket of figs as well, a request that was granted by the guards. Soon after, she sent messengers to Octavian indicating that she wanted to be buried alongside Anthony. Cleopatra was subsequently found dead by Octavian and his men. The specific mysterious circumstances surrounding her actual death continue to intrigue historians even today. Plutarch said, "The messengers came at full speed, and found the guards apprehensive of nothing; but on opening the doors they saw her stone dead, lying upon a bed of gold, set out in all her royal ornaments." Her son Caesarion, possible offspring of Caesar, was later executed, supposedly by order of Octavian [3].

2.2 CLEOPATRA'S REIGN. HER DOWNFALL AND HER DEATH

The queen of all queens, Cleopatra VII, was enthroned as queen of the Ptolemaic Dynasty and Pharaoh of Egypt, inheriting, apart from the Crown, the great inclination of the Ptolemies toward medicine and their love for science. Despite the fact that she reigned during politically turbulent times, she managed to acquire at least some rudimentary knowledge of medicine. She was aware of gynecological diseases and was conversant in pharmacology and botany, and may have authored several scientific texts. Some essays were found beside her head in her tomb but are no longer extant. She produced her own eye makeup, aromatic oils, remedies for baldness, antiseptics, and beauty products [7–8]. She wrote a treatise called the "Cosmetics," which discussed remedies, potions, and ointments. This treatise was mentioned by Galen (third century), Aëtius of Amida in Alexandria (sixth century), Paul of Aegina (seventh century), and John Tzetes (twelfth century) [9]. The longevity of this work's usefulness owes a debt to her knowledge of pharmacology and cosmetics.

During Cleopatra's reign, the city of Alexandria was a center of science. Inside the famous Library of Alexandria were 700,000 treatises and manuscripts, works from mainland Greece, the Aegean, Asia Minor, and Pontos, all gathered in an extraordinary assembly. The Alexandrian medical school was famous for advances and instruction in anatomy, physiology, and pharmacology. The knowledge of potions, poisons, and antidotes was so pervasive during that era in Alexandria that philosophers and physicians believed that production could and should be administered by simple pharmacists, so that the philosophers and physicians could focus on the dosage of the drugs and the patient himself. The Greeks introduced the concept of *theriac*, a versatile, multifunctional drug-antidote to cure all diseases. The theriac was composed of a large number of plant, animal, and mineral substances, mixed with a base of viper venom or blood and blood from animals fed with poisonous plants. Mithridates himself invented a theriac named Mithridatiki. It is more than likely that Roman scholars knew about this ultimate potion and that the Egyptians became familiar with it as well. Cleopatra herself gave poisonous potions in various dosages to slaves to test its toxic limits [10].

Cleopatra was, in fact, a neglected child who wasn't meant to rule. She was well educated and fluent in seven languages, including Egyptian, unlike the rest of the royal family. She lived in a competitive environment, full of conspiracies, intrigues, murders, revolts, civil wars, and infidelity. Her only weapon for survival was to believe in herself. She was forced to marry her young brother, to battle against her family, to deal with the Roman invasion, and to counterplot against her ministers. Over time, she developed a narcissistic personality, a strong character to withstand obstacles, and a complex emotional fabric that could brook no defeat, a difficult mask to uphold [3,11]. Paying great attention to cosmetics and personal charm, she became an example of the perfect *femme fatale* whose technique for ruling was to control the minds and hearts of the vigorous governors of the era [3].

The circumstances surrounding her death are still cloaked in mystery. First off, did she commit suicide or was she murdered? Three possible scenarios need to be considered:

   i. suicide by poison (possibly hidden somewhere in her mausoleum),
  ii. suicide by the venom of the Egyptian cobra, usually referred to as an asp, or viper, or
 iii. poisoning by Octavian and/or his men [12].

No written documents were found to divulge the secret. The oldest reference was that of Strabo (64/63 BC–c. 24 AD), who mentioned that her death could have been the result of a toxic poison or the bite of an asp, so that it was not clear whether it was a murder or suicide [13]. Cleopatra's physician, Olympus, came to almost the same conclusion, except to emphasize that if poison was taken, it was as an ointment administered dermally, rather than a potion swallowed, a fact that increases the certainty that Cleopatra was an expert in the field, cognizant of drugs in their different formulations [12].

Considering the two indistinct prick marks on her body, Galen theorized that she broke the skin by biting her own arm [14]. Thus, several death scene scenarios are:

   i. The skin marks were self-inflicted. This is the less likely scenario, though, for a woman so devoted to her own beauty [10]. She could, instead, have committed suicide simply by swallowing the proper dose of poison.

ii. The marks were made by Mark Anthony when dying in her arms. Realizing Cleopatra's lies and her role in having him take his own life, he could have bitten her in vengeance [3]. This could have happened if we see Mark Anthony as an angry, betrayed, and deceived emperor of the East Roman empire, and a victim of Cleopatra's charms.
iii. The marks were made by instruments used by Cleopatra's maids, or her eunuch, or by Octavian's men to apply the poison by penetrating the skin. Because of her revulsion for pain and bodily imperfections, this would have been undertaken by force.
iv. The marks were actually made by a snakebite, a less likely scenario.

Cleopatra had a deep understanding of poisons [8], as well as a personal physician trained in the Alexandrian School [12], and almost certainly possessed an apothecary of potions, poisons, and antidotes. Along with the poison, Cleopatra might have been able to take a drug to reduce the suffering. She might, as well, have developed a partial immunity to common poisons if she had been regularly self-administering a theriac. If this were the case, she may have required a more potent poison to successfully achieve suicide. Psychologically, Cleopatra saw herself as the woman who had almost magically controlled both Caesar and Mark Anthony, and must have felt that she could do the same with Octavian, albeit without seduction as the outcome. Thus, it is reasonable to assume that she was primed to take the situation in hand and would not have sacrificed her ego by giving in to Octavian.

Cleopatra was permitted by Octavian to conduct Mark Anthony's burial rites. It is possible that when she and her retinue were returning to the royal palace, someone had brought one or more snakes inside the walls. Later, she prepared a feast and asked for a royal bath before sitting down to her meal. She had ordered some figs, which presented a second opportunity for snakes to be smuggled into her quarters, unnoticed by the guards [3]. Soon after Cleopatra's death, the tale of its being caused by a snakebite became an accepted myth in Rome [3,15−16] (Figure 2.2). But was a eunuch or maid strong enough to carry a basket or water jug filled with large and heavy Royal Cobras (each averaging 3−4 m, or 9.8−13 ft, length and weighing some 6 kg or 13 lbs), and camouflaged by figs? It is difficult to confirm this course of events.

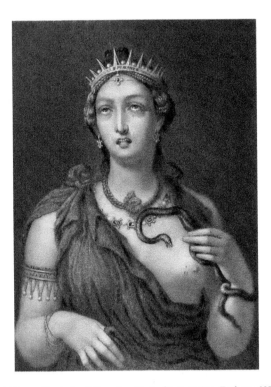

Figure 2.2 Jean-André Rixens. The death of Cleopatra. Musée des Augustins, Toulouse, 1874.

More than one snake might have been needed because two of Cleopatra's handmaidens, Iras and Charmion, were also found dead. Curiously, there were no reports of shouts which might have been caused by pain, nor was swelling of the victim's body noted by the guards or Cleopatra's physician [12]. The vipers' hemotoxic venom causes subcutaneous and intestinal hemorrhage, resulting in a brutal death. Both cobra and viper venom kill after 2—4 and 6—12 h, respectively, quite a long time frame, as Strabo points out. Three women, Cleopatra, Iras, and Charmion, had died within a few minutes, from something which left no physical or pathological marks [17]. Cleopatra, according to the snake poisoning theory, would have been bitten by the serpent, and after the envenomation would have had to be physically and emotionally capable of handing it, if a single snake, to her handmaiden, who, after receiving her own mortal bite, would hand it over, in turn, to the other handmaiden and/or to the eunuch. This scenario does not seem plausible even though a large Egyptian cobra is capable of inflicting a quick death with inconspicuous marks [3]. The fact that only 22—30% of snakebite victims die after African cobra or viper envenomation [18–19] again argues against the likelihood of such a death for Cleopatra and her maids. We may also question where so large a snake or snakes quickly disappeared to, as Octavian and his men supposedly rushed to Cleopatra's windowless and sealed mausoleum. In fact, they arrived so quickly that the second handmaiden was still alive [10]. Moreover, Octavian was familiar with Cleopatra's cunning and dexterous movements and had her heavily guarded [3,17]. This leads us to the final possible scenario: her murder by the ambitious and resourceful Octavian himself.

Octavian knew that his future would be more secure if he could totally remove Cleopatra and her political influence from Egypt. He understood that even if she were imprisoned, she would still pose a danger either by fomenting an outright revolt or by charming the next Roman ruler of the Egyptian province. If Octavian had chosen a public lynching or other humiliation, he would have diminished the nobility of Cleopatra as a mighty and royal queen, and he would have been seen as a strict, vindictive tyrant. Thus, for Octavian one way in particular would have held a great appeal: an injection of one of various poisons which would provide a quick and relatively painless death [3]. The Roman legions, during their campaigns, traveled with their personal physicians [19]. A mixture of poisons, say of hemlock, opium, and aconite, could induce a deep sleep resulting in coma and death [20]. Octavian and his men might have injected Cleopatra with an instrument which would make it appear that she had been bitten by a snake. Cleopatra was a revered queen for most Egyptians. Death from the sacred Egyptian Royal Cobra might have been deemed almost romantic. Octavian had ample time to eliminate all evidence and fabricate a convincing story of whatever death scene he chose. He had both the motive, that is, to permanently remove the political threat of Cleopatra, and the know-how and time to murder her. The subsequent murder of Caesarion, the politically threatening offspring of Cleopatra and Julius Caesar, further strengthens the plausibility that she was murdered [10].

2.3 EPILOGUE

Cleopatra VII, Pharaoh of the Egyptians [8], ruler of the Egyptian empire, whisperer of powerful men, charming, well-educated, and a strong woman, died relatively young. Although we may never know for certain, the preponderance of evidence seems to suggest that rather than committing suicide with an asp, she was murdered. A proponent of Egyptian independence, for which she fought but which battle she lost, she became a victim of politics. Octavian quite possibly had her killed with a poisonous concoction, and to avoid turmoil in the streets of Egypt, presented the world with a trumped-up story about her suicide. After Cleopatra's demise, Octavian became known as Pharaoh. He was given unprecedented powers and named Augustus by the Senate. The Roman Republic became the Roman Empire, and Octavian was its first Emperor.

REFERENCES

[1] Heather P. The great library of Alexandria? San Diego, CA: Library Philosophy and Practice; 2010.

[2] Dimitsas M. History of Alexandria. Athens: Palamidis; 1885.

[3] Burstein SM. The reign of Cleopatra. London: Greenwood Press; 2004.

[4] Seppard S. Pharsalus 48 BC, Caesar and Pompey, clash of the titans. Oxford: Osprey Publishing Ltd; 2006.

[5] Roller DR. Cleopatra, a biography. New York, NY: Oxford University Press; 2010.

[6] Maloney W. The death of Cleopatra, a medical analysis of the theory of suicide by Naja haje. WebmedCentral Toxicol 2010;8:WMC00502.

[7] Caesar GJ, Gardner JF. Caesar, the civil war. New York, NY: Penguin Books; 1967.

[8] Tsoucalas G, Kousoulis AA, Poulakou-Rebelakou E, Karamanou M, Papagrigoriou-Theodoridou M, Androutsos G. Queen Cleopatra and the other "Cleopatras": their medical legacy. J Med Biogr 2013. Available from: http://dx.doi.org/doi:10.1177/0967772013480602.

[9] Skevos Z. War Kleopatra von Aegypten ein Arzt? [Was Cleopatra of Egypt a doctor?]. In: Bohn DHF, editor. Janus, vol. III. Haarlem: Archives internationales pour l' Histoire de la Médecine; 1902.

[10] Plat IM. Women writers of ancient Greece and Rome. Chippenham: Anthony Rowe Ltd; 2004.

[11] Tsoukalas I. Paediatrics from Homer until today. Thessaloniki–Skopelos: Science Press; 2004.

[12] Orland RM, Orland FJ, Orland PT. Psychiatric assessment of Cleopatra: a challenging evaluation. Psychopathology 1990;23(3):169–75.

[13] Strabo. The geography of Strabo (Jones HL, editor). London: Harvard University Press–William Heinemann Ltd; 1924.

[14] Galen. De theriaca ad pisonem [Kunh, CG, Trans.]. In: Claudii Galeni opera omnia. Hildesheim: G. Olms; 1964–1965.

[15] Vergilius PM. Aeneis, Book VIII. Paris: Delalain; 1825.

[16] Horatius FQ. Odes, Book I. Athens: Dimitrakos; 1912.

[17] Guillemain B. Mort de Cléopâtre. Hist Sci Med 2009;43(4):369–73.

[18] Espinoza R. In relation to Cleopatra and snake bites. Rev Med Chil 2001;129(10):1222–6.

[19] Davies R. Service in the Roman army. Edinburgh: Edinburgh University Press; 1989.

[20] Mihailidis C. How Cleopatra died? Athens: Eleyterotypia Tegopoulos; 2010.

CHAPTER 3

Mithridates of Pontus and His Universal Antidote

Adrienne Mayor

Mithridates VI Eupator of Pontus inherited the small, wealthy kingdom of Pontus on the Black Sea (today northeastern Turkey) in 120 BC, after his father was poisoned by enemies. With good reason to believe that his mother, Queen Laodice, intended to poison him in order to control Pontus, the teenaged Mithridates went into hiding for several years. Upon his return he assumed his throne and used poison (likely arsenic) to eliminate several treacherous relatives and rivals. Mithridates, who claimed descent from Persian royalty and Alexander the Great, became the most dangerous and relentless enemy of the late Roman Republic in decades-long conflicts known as the Mithridatic Wars. After his defeat by Pompey in the Third Mithridatic War, he was forced to commit suicide (63 BC).

Driven by his fears of assassination by poison, Mithridates is acknowledged as the first experimental toxicologist, carrying out proto-scientific experiments with poisons and antidotes [1]. His goal was to create a "universal antidote" to make himself and his friends immune to all poisons and toxins. An erudite scholar in many tongues, he had access to myriad poisons, toxicological traditions, and examples, both mythic and historical, to guide him [2].

3.1 INFLUENCES

Mithridates was aware that his land was the home of the mythical witch Medea, adept in poisons and magic. Medea was said to tame unquenchable flames from the petroleum pools of Baku on the Caspian Sea, and her potions were said to bestow superhuman powers, deathlike sleep, or immunity from fire or sword. She also knew the secrets of deadly "dragon's blood" (a name for the toxic mineral realgar) and all the antidotes for serpent venom, secrets eagerly sought by young Mithridates, future toxicologist [2].

History of Toxicology and Environmental Health. DOI: http://dx.doi.org/10.1016/B978-0-12-800045-8.00004-6

Mithridates' own grandfather, King Pharnaces I of Pontus, was credited with the discovery of a "panacea" (cure-all, centaury plant, Pliny 25.79). Another probable influence would have been the unusual research first begun by "mad" Attalus III of Pergamon, the last king of a neighboring land taken over by Mithridates during his conquests of Asia Minor. Pergamon, with its great library, active scientific community, and the healing temple of Asclepius, was the center of medical learning. Nicander of Colophon, a Greek physician who wrote the *Theriaca* on venomous creatures, and the *Alexipharmaka* on poisons and antidotes, was a member of Attalus's court [3]. Ancient and modern historians have assumed that the eccentric King Attalus was insane because he preferred scientific experimentation to governing. As a boy, Mithridates heard the rumors accusing Attalus of poisoning his relatives and foes and mocking him for withdrawing from court life, devoting himself to tending his extensive gardens, and studying botany, pharmacology, and metallurgy. He died in 133 BC, around the time of Mithridates' birth [1,4].

But was Attalus really insane? Modern historian Kent Rigsby suggests that the king's reputation for murder and madness was perpetuated by those who wanted to make Attalus seem an unfit ruler. Pointing out that scientific and philosophical pursuits were typical of several other sophisticated Hellenistic monarchs, Rigsby reasons that that "in reality, Attalus was a scientist and scholar." Attalus may have been eccentric, but his activities seem to constitute scientific research [5].

Indeed, the most remarkable significance of Attalus's research for understanding Mithridates has been overlooked by Rigsby and other modern historians. Justin's most damning example (36.4) of Attalus's insanity was the king's obsession with "digging and sowing in his garden" and his bizarre practice of concocting "mixtures of both healthful and beneficial plants and drenching them with the juices of poisonous ones." Attalus presented these concoctions as "special gifts to his friends." Ancient historians (Plutarch *Demetrius* 20.2; Diodorus 34−35.3) tell us that Attalus cultivated toxic plants such as "henbane, hellebore, hemlock, aconite (monkshood), and thorn apple (*Datura*) in his royal gardens and became an expert in their juices and fruits." The celebrated physician from Pergamon, Galen (b. AD 129), added further information. Galen said that Attalus experimented with antidotes against the venoms of snakes, spiders, scorpions, and toxic sea slugs. Galen (*Antidotes* 1.1) praised Attalus for testing his mixtures only on condemned criminals [3].

It can be no coincidence that Mithridates engaged in the very same sorts of activities and experiments as his own grandfather Pharnaces, "mad" King Attalus, and Nicolas of Colophon. According to Justin, Mithridates began his investigations of *pharmaka* (ancient Greek for drug or medicine) as a boy, secretly testing toxins and antidotes on others and himself. Mithridates' celebrated "universal antidote," an alexipharmic panacea or theriac that later came to be known as the *Mithridatium*, was created by mixing minuscule doses of deadly poisons with antidotes [2].

As king, Mithridates was known to have "amassed detailed knowledge from all his subjects, who covered a substantial part of the world" (Aelian *On Animals* 9.29). His international library of ethnobotanical and toxicological treatises described drugs used by the Druids of Gaul and Mesopotamian doctors, and he could have studied the works of Hindu Ayurvedic ("long-life") practitioners, such as the antidote recipe of Sushruta (ca. 550 BC), which boasted 85 ingredients, and the *Mahagandhahasti* theriac of Charaka (300 BC), which had 60. In 88 BC, Mithridates received Marsi envoys from Italy, shamans known for their *pharmaka* based on venoms. Mithridates likely studied the alchemical writings of Democritus of Egypt, drawing on those of King Menes, who had cultivated poisonous and medicinal plants in 3000 BC. Mithridates corresponded with the doctor Zopyrus in Egypt, who shared his "universal remedy" of 20 ingredients. Another scientific colleague was Asclepiades of Bithynia, who founded an influential medical school in Rome. He declined Mithridates' invitation to work in Sinope but dedicated treatises to the king and sent him antidote formulas [2].

3.2 PHARMACOLOGICAL AND TOXIC RICHES

Natural resources with powerful healthful or noxious characteristics abounded in the Black Sea region. There were many venomous snakes, for example. Mithridates' allies on the steppes, the mounted nomad archers of Scythia, poisoned their arrows with a sophisticated concoction of viper venom and other pathogens. Scythian shamans, called Agari, were experts in antidotes based on venoms, and several Agari joined Mithridates' investigations. Mithridates and other experimenters of his day were well aware of the thin line that divided potentially lethal doses from potentially beneficial amounts of powerful agents.

His Agari doctors saved Mithridates' life on the battlefield by using snake venom to stop severe bleeding from a thigh wound, a medical milestone in the use of venom beneficially. Today, tiny amounts of viper venom from the Caucasus are used to staunch uncontrollable hemorrhage and investigators are creating anticancer drugs from venoms.

Mithridates' ally to the east, Armenia, had remote lakes with venomous fish. His birthplace of Pontus boasted its own extraordinary flora and fauna [6]. Wild honey, distilled by bees from the nectar of poisonous rhododendrons and oleander so profuse on the Black Sea coast, contained a deadly neurotoxin. Even the flesh of Pontic ducks was poisonous. The ducks thrived on hellebore and other baneful plants, and the bees enjoyed a strange immunity to poison. These mysterious natural facts may have inspired Mithridates to search for ways to protect himself from poisons. Beavers were another prized Pontic product; their testicles were valued for treating fever and boosting immunity and sexual vigor, and in perfumes. Castoreum, from beaver musk glands, does contain salicylic acid, the active ingredient in aspirin, derived from willow bark, the beavers' chief food [2].

The kingdom of Pontus was blessed with rich sources of *pharmaka*, potent substances and products used in many different technologies and crafts such as metal working, dyes, and pigments; in making medicines, unguents, and perfumes; and as poisons. Mithridates' extensive Black Sea Empire possessed myriad toxic plants, used for beneficial drugs or poisons: henbane, yew, belladonna or deadly nightshade, hemlock, thorn apple, monkshood, hellebore, poppies, fly agaric mushrooms, rhododendron, and oleander, to name a few [2].

Nefarious, rare substances were mined in Mithridates' lands, from plentiful deposits of gold, silver, copper, iron, rock salt, mercury, sulfur, arsenic, and petroleum, among other rare and potentially dangerous substances [6]. Sinope, the capital of Pontus, was the center for processing and exporting Sinopic red earth, realgar, orpiment, and other glittering dark red and yellow crystals surrounded by magical and ominous folklore in antiquity. Known by many different names, these minerals occurred in association with quicksilver (mercury), lead, sulfur, iron ore, cobalt, nickel, and gold excavated in Pontus; Armenia was known for arsenic mines. These mines exhaled vapors so noxious that they were worked by slaves who had been sentenced to death for crimes. One of the most infamous mines of Mithridates' kingdom was Sandarakurgion Dag (Mount Realgar), on the Halys River. According to the ancient geographer Strabo (11.14.9; 12.3.40–41), gangs of 200 slaves at a time labored to hollow out the entire mountain. Mount Realgar Mine was finally abandoned as unprofitable, because it was too expensive to continually replace the slaves as they dropped dead from the toxic fumes.

The ancient terms for these groups of related compounds make them difficult to identify today. *Cinnabar, zinjifrah, vermilion, Sinopic red earth, ruby sulfur, sinople, orpiment, oker, sandaracha, sandyx, zamikh, arsenicum, Armenian calche, realgar, dragon's blood*: these were ancient names for the many forms of toxic ores containing mercury, sulfur, and/or arsenic. Sinopic red earth was used to waterproof ships; many of these costly substances were prized as brilliant pigments, varnishes, and textile dyes; they were also important in alchemy and medicine. Arsenic (from ancient Persian *zamikh*, "yellow orpiment") is an odorless poison undetectable in food or drink—the ideal toxin for murder (toxic minerals known in antiquity, Pliny 33.31.98; 33.32.99–100; 33.36–41; 35.13–15; 34.55–56.178; Theophrastus on Stones 8.48–60). The poison that someone slipped into Mithridates' father's meat or wine and that Mithridates used to get rid of enemies was most likely pure arsenic, produced by heating realgar (*rhaj al ghar*, Arabic, "powder of the mine"), red arsenic sulfate.

3.3 AVOIDING ASSASSINATION BY POISON

Mithridates undertook many precautions against assassination by poison. There were guards in his kitchens as well as royal tasters. He knew that some metals and certain crystals and stones were believed to detect—even neutralize—poison in food or drink. Mithridates would have owned so-called "poison cups," goblets made of electrum, a gold and silver alloy. A vessel of electrum was said to reveal the presence of poison when iridescent colors rippled across the metallic surface with a crackling sound, apparently the result of a chemical reaction (Pliny 25.5–7, 33.23.81, 37.15.55–61). Other objects, such as amber, red coral, and *glossopetra* ("tongue stones"), were reputed to magically deflect poisons. Tongue stones were actually fossilized giant shark teeth taken from limestone deposits. On contact with poison, these objects reportedly would "sweat" or change color. The shark teeth could also be ground into a powder that deactivated poison. In fact, calcium carbonate in fossils does react with arsenic through *chelation*, a chemical process in which the calcium carbonate mops up the arsenic molecules [7].

Mithridates tested the nature of poisons for other reasons besides ensuring his own immunity. He also sought to learn which poisons were best for undetectable assassinations of enemies and which poisons were ideal for suicide. According to several sources, Mithridates carried suicide pills and distributed them to his commanders and friends. Those capsules, concealed in rings, amulets, and the hilts of daggers and swords, obviously would have contained a fast-acting, relatively gentle, lethal poison with no known antidote (Pliny 33.5.15, 33.6.25–26; Plutarch *Pompey* 32).

Mithridates' chief toxicological coinvestigator was the Greek "root-cutter" (botanist) named Krateuas. In the course of their systematic study of the effects of common and rare *pharmaka*, Mithridates discovered a curious phenomenon. By ingesting tiny amounts of arsenic each day, he achieved an immunity to larger, otherwise fatal doses. Apparently he achieved tolerance to arsenic as a youth, since sources tell us that conspirators in the palace failed in their attempts to poison him while he was a boy. As king, Mithridates liked to exhibit his remarkable ability to dine safely on poison-laced meat and wine, fatal to others (Aulus Gellius 17). Such theatrical demonstrations enhanced the king's reputation of invincibility. Mithridates was said to follow the "ethical" approach of King Attalus praised by Galen, by experimenting only on himself and condemned criminals [3]. In one instance, Mithridates received an envoy with a letter and package from his friend Zopyrus in Alexandria. The letter informed Mithridates that the messenger had been sentenced to death and invited the king to test the accompanying antidote on him [4]. The imagined reactions of the courtiers and foreign dignitaries present at Mithridates' sensational demonstrations of immunity inspired A.E. Housman's poem ("Terence, This Is Stupid Stuff," in *A Shropshire Lad*, 1896): "I tell the tale that I heard told. Mithridates, he died old."

Mithridates' mastery of poisons and his unusually long life is memorialized in the term *mithridatism*, the practice of systematically ingesting small doses of deadly substances to make oneself immune to them. With some toxins, the process can be effective. It is possible to acquire tolerance for levels of arsenic that would kill others, for example. It was observed in antiquity that people of North Africa were less affected by local venomous insects and scorpions (*Aelian On Animals* 5.14; 9.29). Mithridates also understood the little-known fact that snake venom can be safely digested if swallowed—it is only deadly if it enters the bloodstream. The rising incidence of poisoning in the Roman Empire inspired the Roman satirist Juvenal to joke that murder weapons of "cold steel might make a comeback if people would take a hint from old Mithridates and sample the pharmacopeia till they are invulnerable to every drug." [6]

3.4 THE SECRET ANTIDOTE

In antiquity, each natural poison—animal, plant, or mineral—was believed to have a natural antidote. Traditional theriacs normally combined substances that were thought to counter poisons (Pliny 25.2.5–8). Mithridates' basic recipe probably contained some of those common ingredients, such as cinnamon, myrrh, cassia, honey, castor, musk, frankincense, rue, tannin, garlic, Lemnian earth, Chian wine, charcoal, curdled milk, centaury, aristolochia (birthwort), ginger, iris (orris root), rue, *Eupatorium*, rhubarb, hypericum (St. John's wort), saffron, walnuts, figs, parsley, acacia, carrot, cardamom, anise, opium, and other ingredients from the Mediterranean and Black Sea, Arabia, North Africa, Eurasia, and India [2,4]. Modern science reveals that some of these substances can counteract illness and toxins. For example, the sulfur in garlic neutralizes arsenic in the bloodstream. Charcoal absorbs and filters many different toxins. Garlic, myrrh, cinnamon, and St. John's wort are antibacterial. Recent studies of many common *Mithridatium* ingredients reveal bioactivities in the immune system. Certain plants long used by folk healers in Africa and India neutralize cobra, adder, and viper venoms [2].

Mithridates' personal theriac or tonic was special because it combined *both* toxic *and* beneficial *pharmaka*. Building on the work begun by Attalus III, Nicander of Colophon, and others, Mithridates recorded the properties of hundreds of poisons and antidotes in experiments on prisoners, associates, and himself. "Through tireless research and every possible experiment," wrote Pliny, Mithridates sought ways to "compel poisons to be helpful remedies." Mithridates and Krateuas, joined by the physician Papias, Persian Magi and Scythian Agari healers, and Timotheus, a specialist in war wounds, tested many health-giving essences compounded with minute amounts of poisons. They created an *electuary*, a paste held together with honey and molded into a large pill. Mithridates reportedly ingested his secret theriac with cold spring water on a daily basis (Pliny 25.6−7; 25.17.37; 25.26.62−63; 25.29.65). Apparently the concoction was harmless and may have promoted his immune system. The ancient sources agree that Mithridates enjoyed robust health into his 70s, at a time when the average lifespan was 45 [1,2].

After his death, Mithridates' personal library and archives were taken to Rome and translated into Latin by Lenaeus (95−25 BC). Pliny (25.2.5−8; 25.79−82) studied Mithridates' private papers and concluded, "We know from direct evidence and by report" that Mithridates "was a more accomplished researcher into biology than any man before him. In order to become immune to poison by making his body accustomed to it, he alone devised the plan to drink poison every day, after first taking remedies."

The key principle of Mithridates' theriac was the combination of beneficial drugs and antitoxins with tiny amounts of poisons, the approach followed by Attalus and Hindu doctors. Myriad poisons were known in antiquity, from viper, scorpion, and jellyfish venoms to the deadly sap of yew trees and the crimson crystals of cinnabar [6]. Pliny described about 7000 venific substances in his encyclopedia of natural history and he listed numerous plants, some with powerful, even dangerous, bioactive properties that were said to counter them, such as scordion, fly agaric mushrooms, artemesia, centaury, polemonia, and aristolochia. Arsenic—the notorious "powder of succession" in antiquity—would have been the first poison Mithridates sought to defend against. Arsenic interferes with essential proteins for metabolism. In small doses, however, enzymes produced by the liver bind to and inactivate arsenic. Taking small amounts over time causes the liver to produce more enzymes, allowing one to survive a normally lethal dose. Mithridates was essentially investigating whether a similar process might work with plant poisons. Mithridates had observed natural tolerances to poisonous plants in rats, insects, birds, and other creatures. According to Pliny and Aulus Gellius (17), the poison blood of Pontic ducks was included in the *Mithridatium* [4]. It is now known that some species of ducks and other birds do eat poison hemlock without harm. Because they do not excrete the toxic alkaloids, their blood and flesh becomes poisonous without harm to them but dangerous to those who eat them [2].

What other poisons were included in the original *Mithridatium*? Perhaps toxic honey from Pontus—in tiny amounts it was considered a tonic (Aelian *On Animals* 5.4). Various reptiles—such as toxic skinks, salamanders, and vipers—were also said to be part of Mithridates' recipe, based on the notion that all poisonous creatures must produce antidotes to their own toxins in their bodies. Modern scientific experiments show that nonfatal doses of snake venom can stimulate the immune response and allow humans to withstand up to 10 times the amount of venom that would be fatal without inoculation. A similar process works with some insect stings and a variety of toxins. Surprising scientific studies of a "counterintuitive" process called *hormesis* show that very low doses of certain toxins activate a protective mechanism, so that when a larger dose is encountered, it is not as damaging. According to this new concept—remarkably akin to Mithridates' own hypothesis 2000 years ago—minute doses of poison substances can be analogous to a vaccine [2].

Could the unusual properties of St. John's wort, *hypericum*, listed in many *Mithridatium* recipes, help to solve the ancient riddle of Mithridates' immunity? Molecular scientists have recently discovered hypericum's remarkable antidote effect, not yet completely understood. The herb activates the liver to produce a potent enzyme that is capable of neutralizing a great many potentially dangerous chemicals—as well as prescribed drugs for various conditions. If St. John's wort was included in Mithridates' antidote, it would have stimulated what could be called a hypervigilant "chemical surveillance system" with the capacity to sense and break down normally fatal doses of many different toxins [2].

3.5 MITHRIDATIUM'S LEGACY

After Mithridates' death, several imperial doctors in Rome claimed to know the secret *Mithridatium* formula. Poisonings and fears of poisoning were commonplace in the Roman Empire. "If you want to survive to gather rosebuds for another day," commented Juvenal (14.251−55), "find a doctor to prescribe some of the drug that Mithridates invented. Before every meal take a dose of the stuff that saves kings" [6].

Was it possible that Mithridates' genuine recipe was known by some in Rome? Perhaps Mithridates entrusted the secret to his friend Asclepiades, the most famous doctor in Rome [4]. According to Galen (*Opera Omnia* 14; *Antidotes* 2), a doctor named Aelius reportedly prescribed *Mithridatium* for Julius Caesar, who was campaigning in Pontus only 16 years after Mithridates' death [2].

The discovery of an inscription near the Appian Way from the time of Emperor Augustus (b. 63 BC, the year of Mithridates' death) is intriguing. It describes L. Lutatius Paccius (a non-Roman name) as an "incense-seller from the family of King Mithridates." Was he a freed slave? Was he really a relative of Mithridates? Like other ancient apothecaries, Paccius was probably more than just a purveyor of "incense"—why else would he advertise his relationship to Mithridates? Poisons had been strictly regulated since the dictator Sulla's legislation during the Mithridatic Wars. That may explain why an apothecary might only advertise aromatics for sale publicly. Some members of Mithridates' family and his friends did end up in Italy after his death. The inscription suggests that Paccius may have been one of those claiming to know the original *Mithridatium* recipe and that he sold this legendary "trademark" antidote in Rome. A different Paccius, presumably this man's son, later became very rich from selling a very special secret medicine in Rome. This Paccius the Younger bequeathed the "Paccius family recipe" to the Emperor Tiberius, Augustus's successor, in AD 14, according to the famous imperial doctor Celsius [4].

Could that mysterious Paccius "family recipe" have been the basis for the later imperial Roman formulas? Many doctors claimed to have improved Mithridates' original, for example, the version compounded by the imperial doctor Andromachus for the Emperor Nero. Andromachus's *Mithridatium* had 64 ingredients; he replaced minced lizards with venomous snakes and added opium poppy seeds [1]. In 2000, Italian archeologists made a notable discovery at a villa near Pompeii (AD 79). A large vat contained residue consisting of reptile remains and several medicinal plants, including opium poppy seeds. The archeologists suggested that the vat might have been used to prepare Andromachus's version of the legendary *Mithridatium* [2].

Nero died in AD 68, and every Roman emperor thereafter gulped down daily what his personal doctor insisted was a variation based on

Mithridates' original antidote. As the number of "authentic" recipes multiplied, more and more exotic, expensive ingredients were added (Pliny 25.3, 29.8.24–26). A century after Mithridates' death, the physician Celsius mixed 36 ingredients in a concoction that weighed almost 3 pounds, for 6 months' worth of pills to be swallowed with wine. In AD 170, Galen prescribed a liquid *Mithridatium* for Emperor Marcus Aurelius; Galen had added more opium and a fine vintage wine. The wine improved the flavor and the opium certainly guaranteed that the emperor would drink his medicine every day. Later medieval recipes contained as many as 184 ingredients [1].

In ancient and medieval Islamic toxicology manuscripts, the Arabic theriac (*tiryaq-i-faruq, mithruditus*) and Persian (*daryaq*) recipes followed Mithridates' concept of combining poisons with antidotes. Averroes, the Spanish–Arabic philosopher–physician (b. 1126) wrote a treatise on *tiryaq*. In a veiled allusion to paranoid despots of his day who were obsessed with poisoning, he warned against the prolonged use of theriac by healthy people—cautioning that it "could actually transform human nature into a kind of poison." In AD 667, Islamic ambassadors presented the Tang Dynasty emperor of China with a gift of the *Mithridatium* theriac (in Chinese called *tayeqie, diyejia*). Chinese chronicles described it as a dark red lump the size and shape of a pig's gall bladder. Chinese manuscript illustrations show envoys in Persian-style costume offering these red *Mithridatium* pills as tribute to the emperor [2,8].

From the Middle Ages on in Europe, medicines labeled *Mithridatium* were eagerly purchased. European laws required apothecaries to openly display all the precious, costly ingredients and to mix up the *Mithridatium* outdoors in public squares. For more than two millennia after the death of Mithridates, kings, queens, and nobles from Charlemagne and Alfred the Great to Henry VIII and Queen Elizabeth I ingested some form of *Mithridatium* every day. The royal and aristocratic theriac was kept in ornate gold and pottery apothecary jars, many of them illustrating scenes from the life of Mithridates. Apothecaries sold cheaper varieties of *Mithridatium* to ordinary people, kept in plainer jars. Mithridates' universal antidote became the most popular and longest lived prescription in history. A *Mithridatium* was advertised by a pharmacy in Rome as recently as 1984 [1].

Most of the surviving recipes for theriacs in ancient Latin, Greek, Hebrew, Indian, Arabic, and early Islamic medical writings included a range of plant, animal, and mineral *pharmaka* thought to counteract toxins and disease. Aside from Andromachus's addition of chopped vipers for Nero's antidote, however, most of these theriac recipes did not deliberately include poisons (Dio Cassius 37.13; Celsius *De medicina* 5.23.3). Yet most of the ancient Greek and Latin writers agreed with Pliny that Mithridates achieved immunity to poisons by ingesting deadly substances along with a cocktail of specific or general antidotes. In Pliny's words (25.3−7), Mithridates "thought out the plan of drinking poisons daily, after taking remedies, in order that sheer habit might render the poisons harmless."

We can guess at some of the counteracting drugs that Mithridates was likely to have put in his formula, but his precise method of calibrating minuscule doses of poisons and exactly what they were remains a mystery. He and his team worked in secrecy. His original lost recipe was believed to contain more than 50 ingredients, many of them costly, rare substances from distant lands. The confiscated notes translated after his death in Rome listed only a few commonplace ingredients, with the exception of the blood of Pontic ducks. Pliny (29.8.24−26, 23.77.149) expressed surprise at the lack of any obscure or exotic substances in the Mithridatic notes that he studied. He found one scrap of paper in the king's handwriting that said, "Pound together two dried nuts, two figs, and twenty leaves of rue with a pinch of salt: he who takes this while fasting will be immune to all poison for that day." [1,4]. As Pliny reasonably commented, however, this mundane recipe should not be taken seriously—it could have been a forgery or hoax, or a deliberate red herring.

So what became of the original Mithridatium formula? Perhaps Pliny saw only notes that the emperor allowed him to see. The papers taken to Rome after his death may have recorded only Mithridates' earliest experiments, which had been superseded by successful, more complex experiments whose records did not survive. Mithridates' genuine archives could have been lost, destroyed, or hidden away during the chaos of the Mithridatic Wars. It is even possible that Mithridates' documents may have been encrypted—ancient alchemists often wrote in codes or obscure languages to keep their work secret. Mithridates certainly possessed the linguistic skills; he knew nearly two dozen languages. Were the ingredients of the compound formula somehow divulged to imperial Roman doctors who inherited Mithridates' papers or Paccius's recipe? Were written versions of the perfected formula destroyed on Mithridates' orders? Or were they confided only to his closest friends and allies, such as King Tigranes II of Armenia who, like his son-in-law Mithridates, enjoyed vigorous health and an extremely long life? Perhaps the formula was destroyed when Callistratus, Mithridates' personal secretary, was murdered by Roman soldiers during the wars while carrying important papers. After his defeat of Mithridates in 63 BC, the Roman commander Pompey burned many official papers—he might well have burned some of Mithridates' toxicological archives. Or—as suggested by the historian of medicine Alain Touwaide—maybe Pompey actually obtained the original recipe but kept it secret within his circle [4]. Finally, the instructions for the *Mithridatium* may never have been written down. Perhaps they were recorded only in Mithridates' prodigious memory.

Without new evidence—such as a verifiable, datable recipe from the first century BC preserved in writing, or the discovery of sealed jars of the king's own *Mithridatium* containing identifiable residues of known theriac ingredients, or Mithridates' corpse well-preserved enough to permit hair and bone sampling—we will never know the legendary universal antidote's composition. Yet Mithridates' goal of creating a "universal antidote" lives on. Sergei Popov, a top scientist once employed in the ultrasecret Soviet bioweapons program of the 1980s and 1990s, defected to the United States in 1992. Popov's work now focuses on broad-spectrum biodefenses; in other words, he seeks a "universal" antidote to provide immunity to known biotoxins and "weapons-grade" pathogens. Like the Janus-faced *pharmaka* of the *Mithridatium*, the materials Popov investigates hold the potential for great harm or great good [2].

REFERENCES

[1] Griffin J. Mithridates VI of Pontus, the first experimental toxicologist. Adverse Drug React Acute Poisoning Rev 1995;14:1–6.

[2] Mayor A. The poison king: the life and legend of Mithradates, Rome's deadliest enemy. Princeton, NJ: Princeton University Press; 2010.

[3] Scarborough J. Attalus III of Pergamon: research toxicologist. In: Paper, 27th annual meeting of the Classical Association of South Africa, Cape Town; July 2–5, 2007.

[4] Totelin L. Mithradates' antidote—a pharmacological ghost. Early Sci Med 2004;9:1–19.

[5] Rigsby K. Provincia Asia. Trans Am Philol Assoc 1988;118:123–53.

[6] Cilliers L, Retief F. Poisons, poisonings and the drug trade in ancient Rome. Akroterion 2000;45:88–100.

[7] Zammit-Maempel G. Handbills extolling the virtues of fossil sharks' teeth. J Maltese Stud 1978;7:211–24.

[8] Nappi C. Bolatu's pharmacy: theriac in early modern China. Early Sci Med 2008.

CHAPTER 4

Theriaca Magna: The Glorious Cure-All Remedy

Marianna Karamanou and George Androutsos

4.1 INTRODUCTION

Once upon a time an ambitious king rivaled Rome's expanding domin-ions, creating a Black Sea Empire. Claiming descent from Alexander the Great and Persian Royalties, Mithridates VI Eupator (132–63 BC), king of Pontus in Asia Minor, recruited an ethnically diverse army and tried to create an independent East Empire. While Mithridates was still a child, it was said that his mother poisoned his father (Mithridates V) and that after that she become a vicereine. Afraid that his mother would attempt to kill him and living in constant apprehension of being poisoned by his enemies, Mithridates became obsessed with poisons and tried to develop a tolerance by ingesting small amounts of them daily as well as a mixture of antidotes. Experimenting on criminals and slaves, he was one of the first to systematically study poisons in humans. He also created a general antidote, *Mithridatium*, that con-tained 36 ingredients and was said to protect against any known poi-son. Defeated by the Roman military leader Pompey (106–48 BC) in 63 BC, Mithridates poisoned his wives and children but no poison could kill him. In the end, he had to ask his Gallic mercenary bodyguard to kill him with a sword. His work on pharmacology and toxicology was translated into Latin by Pompeius Lenaeus, a learned freedman of Pompey, and *Mithridatium* entered the Roman world [1].

4.2 THERIAC IN ANTIQUITY

In a period in which poisoning was a traditional political weapon and a typical method of royal succession, polyvalent antidotes such as *alex-ipharmaka* or *theriac* (derived from the Greek *therion*, for wild beast) were highly esteemed. These were supposed to induce immunity according to the principle that like cures like, by gradually introducing small amounts of poison into the organism. Subsequently, several

History of Toxicology and Environmental Health. DOI: http://dx.doi.org/10.1016/B978-0-12-800045-8.00005-8

kinds of theriacs were produced but the most celebrated was perhaps that invented by Adromachus the Elder, a Cretan who became *Archiater* (chief physician) to the Emperor Nero (54–68 CE).

Andromachus's concoction, *Galene Theriaca* (tranquility theriac), was an improved version of Mithridates's elixir, containing 65 ingredients with a higher proportion of opiates and minerals and with the original lizard flesh replaced by that of a viper [2]. The recipe for *Galene* was written in Greek by Andromachus in the form of elegiac couplets and the prose rendition was quoted by his son Andromachus the Younger:

> *Pastils of squill 48 drachms; pastils of viper's flesh 24 drachms; pastils of hedy-chroum and black pepper 24 drachms each; poppy juice 24 drachms; dry roses, water germander, turnip seeds, iris from Illyricum, agaric from Pontus, cinnamon, licorice juice, opobalsam, of each 12 drachms; myrrh, saffron, ginger, rhubarb from Pontus, cinquefoil root, calamint, horehound, parsley, lavender, saussurea lappa, white pepper, long pepper, dittany from Crete, fragrant rush flower, frankincense, turpentine, cassia bark quill, nard from India, of each 6 drachms; germander, ground pine, hypocist, juice of the leaf of white flowered cinnamon, nard from Gaul, gentian root, anise, flesh of lamb from the land of Athamanes, fennel seeds, terra lemnia, roasted copper, cardamon, yellow flag, burnet from Pontus, fruit of balsam-tree, St John's wort, shittah rose, Arabic gum, cardamomum, of each 4 drachms; wild carrot seeds, galbanum, gum from Ferula persica, Hercule's woundwort, bitumen, castoreum, small centaury, small birthwort, of each 2 drachms, of Attic honey 150 drachms; of vetch meal 80 drachms [3] (Figure 4.1).*

The concoction took 40 days to prepare after which the maturation process began. According to Andromachus, his theriac had more applications than simply as a remedy against venomous bites or an antidote for poisons. It was also effective in the treatment of headaches, poor sight, kidney stones, ulcers, dysentery, and deafness; it could induce the menses and dry up the excess of humors in the body (2).

However, almost a century later, another theriac appeared that eclipsed all others in fame and popularity to become a universal panacea. It was the theriac prepared by the distinguished Greek physician Galen (130–c. 201) (Figure 4.2). The basic formula consisted of viper's flesh, opium, honey, and more than 70 other ingredients. Twelve years was considered the proper period to preserve it before use, although the Emperor Marcus Aurelius (121–180 CE) used the mixture within 2 months from its preparation [4]. According to Galen, Marcus Aurelius was taking theriac daily, mixing it with wine or water to protect against poisons and to ensure good health status. This habit,

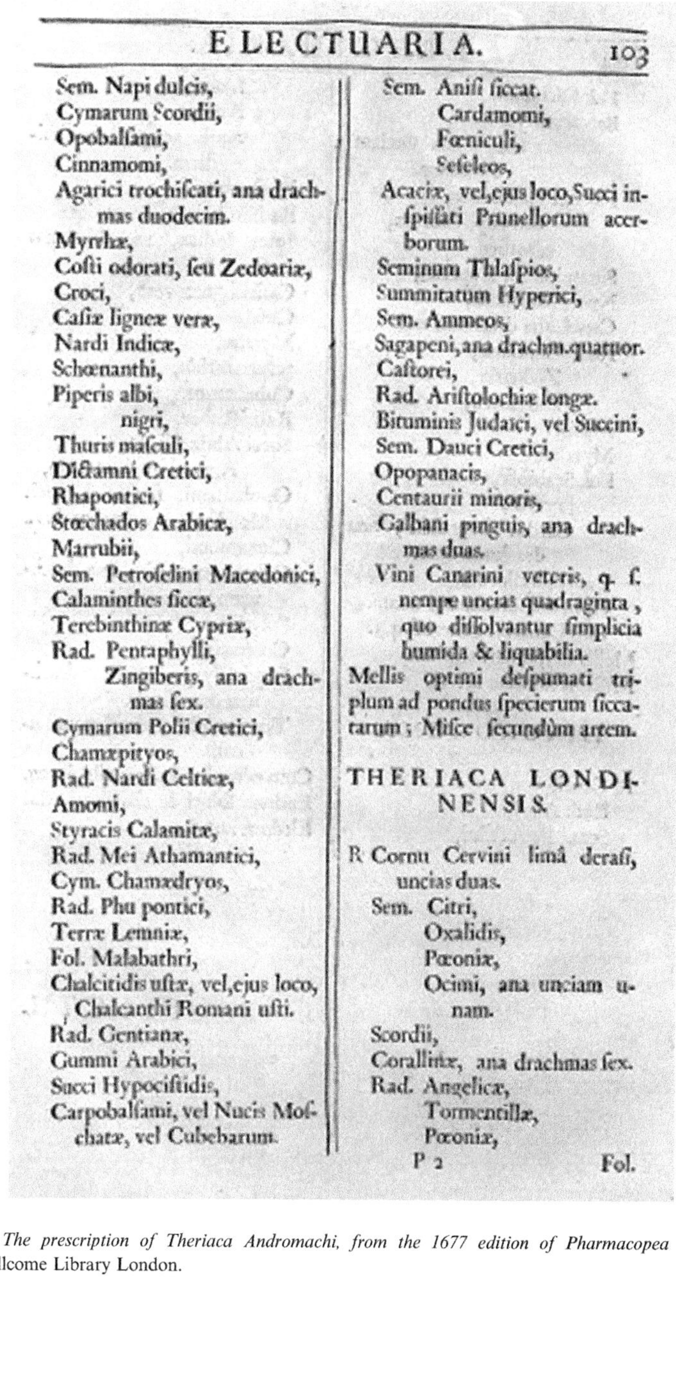

ELECTUARIA.   103

Sem. Napi dulcis,
Cymarum Scordii,
Opobalsami,
Cinnamomi,
Agarici trochiscati, ana drach-
    mas duodecim.
Myrrhæ,
Costi odorati, seu Zedoariæ,
Croci,
Casiæ ligneæ veræ,
Nardi Indicæ,
Schœnanthi,
Piperis albi,
    nigri,
Thuris masculi,
Dictamni Cretici,
Rhapontici,
Stœchados Arabicæ,
Marrubii,
Sem. Petroselini Macedonici,
Calaminthes siccæ,
Terebinthinæ Cypriæ,
Rad. Pentaphylli,
    Zingiberis, ana drach-
    mas sex.
Cymarum Polii Cretici,
Chamæpityos,
Rad. Nardi Celticæ,
Amomi,
Styracis Calamitæ,
Rad. Mei Athamantici,
Cym. Chamædryos,
Rad. Phu pontici,
Terræ Lemniæ,
Fol. Malabathri,
Chalcitidis ustæ, vel,ejus loco,
    Chalcanthi Romani usti.
Rad. Gentianæ,
Gummi Arabici,
Succi Hypocistidis,
Carpobalsami, vel Nucis Mos-
    chatæ, vel Cubebarum.

Sem. Anisi siccat.
Cardamomi,
Fœniculi,
Seseleos,
Acaciæ, vel,ejus loco,Succi in-
    spissati Prunellorum acer-
    borum.
Seminum Thlaspios,
Summitatum Hyperici,
Sem. Ammeos,
Sagapeni, ana drachm.quatuor.
Castorei,
Rad. Aristolochiæ longæ.
Bituminis Judaici, vel Succini,
Sem. Dauci Cretici,
Opopanacis,
Centaurii minoris,
Galbani pinguis, ana drach-
    mas duas.
Vini Canarini veteris, q. s.
    nempe uncias quadraginta ,
    quo dissolvantur simplicia
    humida & liquabilia.
Mellis optimi despumati tri-
plum ad pondus specierum sicca-
tarum ; Misce secundùm artem.

THERIACA LONDI-
NENSIS.

R Cornu Cervini limâ derasi,
    uncias duas.
Sem. Citri,
    Oxalidis,
    Pœoniæ,
    Ocimi, ana unciam u-
    nam.
Scordii,
Corallinæ, ana drachmas sex.
Rad. Angelicæ,
    Tormentillæ,
    Pœoniæ,

P 2   Fol.

Figure 4.1 The prescription of Theriaca Andromachi, from the 1677 edition of Pharmacopea Londinensis.
Source: Wellcome Library London.

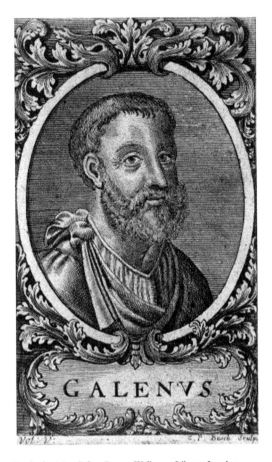

Figure 4.2 The eminent Greek physician Galen. Source: Wellcome Library London.

which influenced his sleep and resulted in a lack of sleep after it was withdrawn, suggests that he was probably addicted to opium [5]. Galen referred to the duration of the drug's efficacy, nowadays known as the expiration date: "Theriac is still effective after thirty years and for all those mild diseases it is recommended even after sixty years. After this span of time, the drug weakens and is no longer effective" [6]. Moreover, Galen experimented with theriac by performing one of the first randomized control trials in history. In his work *De theriaca ad Pisonem* he writes that he took roosters and divided them in two groups. In group A he administered theriac and in group B he did not. Then he brought both groups into contact with snakes. He observed that the roosters of group B died immediately after the bite, while those in group A survived, proving the therapeutic effectiveness of the preparation.

He also mentioned that the above experiment could be used in cases that tested whether theriac was in its natural form or had been adulterated [6].

Galen also reported theriac's therapeutic efficacy on patients: "One of the slaves of the Emperor whose duty was to drive away snakes, having been bitten, took for some time draughts of ordinary medicines, but as his skin changed so as to assume the colour of a leek, he came to me and narrated his accident; after having drunk theriac he recovered quickly his natural colour" [6]. Galen passed his theriac on under the name of *Theriac of Andromachus* and since then its fame as an antidote has led it to be regarded as a cure-all remedy [7].

4.3 THERIAC IN THE MEDIEVAL PERIOD

During the sixth and seventh centuries, theriac is referred to in several passages of the works of Aetius of Amida (502–575 CE) and Paul of Aegina (625–690 CE), while Arabian medicine, under Galenic influence, adopted theriac's use [4,8]. Abulcassis (936–1013 CE) described the preparation of theriac composed of 84 different ingredients, while Maimonides (1135–1204 CE), in his *Treatise on poisons and their antidotes* (1198), noticed the administration of the Great Theriac [9,10]. Avicenna (980–1037 CE) provided an explanation for the medicinal action of theriac which was derived from its specific form, the act of combination and not out of the ingredients, claiming that theriac could not only cure cases of poisoning but could also strengths the heart and preserve the health of a perfectly well man who consumed it regularly [11]. Averroes (1126–1198 CE) held an opposing view: in his treatise on theriac (*Tractatus de tyriaca*), he pointed out that while it was beneficial to the patient as an antidote, it could be dangerous as a regular and repeated medication as it could alter the health status and rendered poisonous. He advised physicians to prescribe it with caution and not as a prophylactic remedy [12].

In the eleventh century, the translation of the works of Arab physicians renewed Western medicine and theriac is listed in its turn among the remedies recommended in the renowned work *Regimen sanitatis* of the Salernian School: "The raddish, pear, theriac, garlic, rue, all potent poisons will at once undo" [13]. In Antidotarium Nicolai (twelfth century), a Salernian collection of some 150 empirical time-tested recipes, theriac is credited with more far-reaching powers of both a therapeutic and a prophylactic nature: "Theriac is good for the most serious afflictions of the human body as epilepsy, catalepsy, headache, stomach ache, migraine, hoarseness, bronchitis, asthma, jaundice, dropsy, leprosy. It induces menstruation and expels the dead fetus. It is especially good against all poisons, and bites. It strengths the heart, brain, liver and keeps the entire body incorrupt" [14].

In the newly founded Montpellier medical school (1221) theriac stimulated keen interest among medical scholars who attempted to determine its mechanism of action and dosage; their work also raised the question of whether it could be administered to the healthy. Arnaud de Villeneuve (1235–1311 CE), Henri de Mondeville (1260–1316 CE), Bernard de Godron (1285–1318 CE), and others relied more or less on Averroes' doctrines, which stated that theriac should not be taken by healthy individuals [15]. In his *Chirugia* (1300), Mondeville mentioned, "It must be noted fifthly that according to Averroes in his book de *Tyriaca*, medicines curing poisons are midway between medicines, the body and poisons; in bloody and choleric illnesses theriac is not of value ... and it should everywhere and always be administered with the greatest precaution while in fevers the use of theriac is almost wholly to be abandoned" [12]. Furthermore, physicians and patients seemed to have been aware of the effects of theriac's ingredients and the fatal consequences of overdosing. Bernard de Gordon was called to treat an apothecary who had accidentally received a fatal dose of theriac: "It happened that a certain apothecary had sold a toxic substance and some remained behind the nail of his thumb. When he began to pick his nose with his thumb, his color began to change and he fainted repeatedly. When he took three drams [of the antidote theriac], his condition became more serious. I was called around midnight and I saw that the amount of theriac had been too high. I made him vomit and after he had purged his stomach sufficiently, I gave him one dram of theriac and he was cured" [16].

Theriac is mentioned in the twelfth-century story of *Tristan and Isolt*. Poisoned by a dragon, Tristan receives care from Isolt: "She felt his body and found that he was still alive; she made him drink some theriac and took such care of him that all of his swelling went down and he was cured and restored to his beauty" [17]. Thanks to the mystique of legend and magic, theriac usage was widespread in the Middle Ages, notably for curing plague. The 1348 *Consultation de la Faculté de Paris* stressed the importance of theriac's administration for plague prophylaxis [18]. In the same way, the notable French surgeon Guy de Chauliac (1300–1368 CE), who witnessed the terrible plague outbreaks of 1358 and 1361, remained healthy thanks to the daily intake of theriac, while several other physicians, among them Johannes Jacobi in his *Regimen contra pestilentiam*, suggested theriac as a cure for and prophylactic remedy against plague [19,20].

4.4 THERIAC IN THE RENAISSANCE

During the Renaissance, theriac became extremely popular and highly prized, taking center stage in the European pharmacopeias, while the ambition to produce a perfect concoction stimulated pharmacists through Europe. The Venetian Republic became the center for the production of the highest-quality theriac known as *Venice treacle*, an official preparation carrying the republic's seal. Its export throughout the rest of Europe provided an important source of revenue [21]. Soon an important question rose: Was the prepared theriac as effective as that of the classical age? There had been cases in which theriac was proved to be ineffective and physicians doubted its action. According to Pietro-Andrea Mattioli (1500–1577 CE), many of the ingredients used in classical times were now unavailable, while Bartolomeo Maranta (d. 1571), author of *Della Theriaca ed del Mithridato*, blamed the ignorance or negligence of physicians and pharmacists for the failure to produce an effective theriac [21]. Concern for guaranteeing the genuineness of the product led the authorities of several cities to supervise its production (Figure 4.3). The manufacturing of theriac in public led to the introduction of strict controls over and standards governing the quality of ingredients, thus stimulating the earliest concepts of medicine regulations.

4.5 CONCLUSION

Kept in ornate porcelain jars, illustrated in scenes from the life of Mithridates, the recipe to produce and to use theriac reached the nineteenth century as it was included in the 1872 German and 1874 French pharmacopeias, and then progressively disappeared [21] (Figure 4.4). Was it a universal antidote or just an addicting tranquilizer, thanks to opium? Either way, its impact on humanity lasted more than 2000 years.

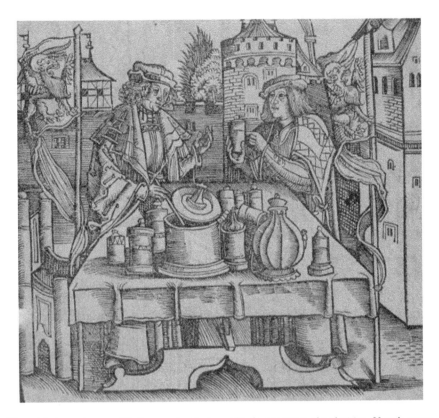

Figure 4.3 An apothecary publically preparing theriac, under the supervision of a physician, fifteenth century.
Source: Wellcome Library London.

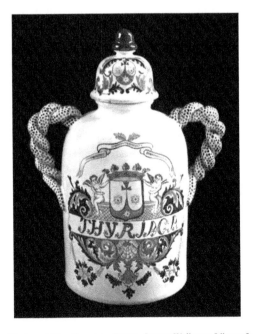

Figure 4.4 Drug jars for Theriac, eighteenth-century France. Source: Wellcome Library London.

REFERENCES

[1] Mayor A. The poison king: the life and legend of Mithradates, Rome's deadliest enemy. Princeton, NJ: Princeton University Press; 2009.

[2] Watson G. Theriac and Mithridatum: a study in therapeutics. London: Wellcome Historical Medical Library; 1966.

[3] Galen. De antidotis I. In: Kühn CG, editor. Claudii galeni opera omnia. Hildesheim: Georg Olms; 1964–5.

[4] Prioreschi PA. History of medicine. Roman medicine, vol. 3. Omaha, NE: Horatius Press; 2001.

[5] Africa TW. The opium addiction of Marcus Aurelius. J Hist Ideas 1961;22:97–102.

[6] Galen. De Theriaca ad Pisonem. In: Kühn XIV CG, editor. Opera omnia. Hildesheim: Georg Olms; 1965.

[7] Karaberopoulos D, Karamanou M, Androutsos G. The *theriac* in antiquity. Lancet 2012;379:1942–3.

[8] Adams F. The medical works of Paulus Aegineta. London: Welsh; 1834.

[9] Hamarneh S, Sonnedecker G. A pharmaceutical view of Abulcasis al Zahrawi. Leiden: Brill; 1963.

[10] Muntner S, editor. The medical writings of Moses Maimonides: treatise on poisons and their antidotes. Philadelphia, PA: J.B. Lippincott Co.; 1966. pp. 57.

[11] Avicenna. The Canon of medicine of Avicenna [Cameron O, Trans.]. NewYork, NY: AMS Press Inc; 1973.

[12] McVaugh MR. Arnaldi de Villanova opera medica omnia. De amore heroico. De dosi tyriacalium medicinarum, vol. 3. Barcelona: Publications de la Universitat de Barcelona; 1985. p. 58–60, 68–70.

[13] Ordronaux J. (Trans.). Regimen sanitatis salerni. Scuola medica salernitana. Philadelphia, PA: Lippincott; 1870.

[14] Grant E, editor. A source book in medieval science. Cambridge, MA: Harvard University Press; 1974. pp. 110.

[15] McVaugh MR. Theriac at Montpellier, 1285–1325 (with an edition of the "Questiones de tyriaca" of William of Brescia). Sudhoffs Arch 1972;56(2):113–44.

[16] Demaitre LE. Doctor Bernard de Gordon: professor and practitioner. Toronto, ON: Pontifical Institute of Mediaeval Studies; 1980.

[17] Spector NB. The Romance of Tristan and Isolt. Evanston, IL: Northwestern University Press; 1973. p. 19.

[18] Michon LAJ, editor. Documents inédits sur la grande peste de 1348 (Consultation de la Faculté de Paris, Consultation d'un practicien de Montpellier, Description de Guillaume de Machaut). Paris: Baillière; 1860.

[19] Jacobi J. Preservatio pestilentie secundum magistrum. Geneva; 1371.

[20] Byrne JP. Encyclopedia of the Black Death. Denver, CO: ABC- CLIO; 2012. p. 72.

[21] Olmi G. In: Zanca A, editor. The prince of all drugs: theriac in pharmacy through ages: ancient drugs. Parma: Farmitalia Carlo Erba; 1990. p. 105–22.

CHAPTER 5

Nicander, *Thêriaka*, and *Alexipharmaka*: Venoms, Poisons, and Literature

Alain Touwaide

The *Thêriaka* and *Alexipharmaka*, by the otherwise not-well-known ancient Greek author Nicander of Colophon, are probably the most paradoxical works in the history of toxicology [1]. They have been transmitted by more than 40 manuscripts—one of which dates as far back as the tenth century and is richly illustrated—with multiple editions, translations, and commentaries by Renaissance physicians and scholars. The first of these was printed in 1499 at the very beginning of Greek scholarly printing, and repeated printed editions by modern Western classicists, including innumerable erudite publications, aimed to decipher the text of these two works.

The *Thêriaka* and *Alexipharmaka* are two poems of 958 and 630 verses, respectively. The former is devoted to venoms and the latter to other poisons. A word of explanation about the use of these words is in order. *Venom* usually refers to a poisonous substance requiring an animal delivery system (for example, snake venoms via biting). On the other hand, *poison* more generally refers to a substance causing harm typically by ingestion, although other routes of exposure, such as absorption through the skin are also possible. Thus, plants such as poison ivy, minerals such as cinnabar (due to its mercury content), and even parts of animals, such as fugu fish, may correctly be called poisons.

The verses of Nicander's two poems reproduce the structure of the *Iliad* and the *Odyssey*, which consists of hexameters. Whatever the exact period of the composition of the *Thêriaka* and *Alexipharmaka* (possibly the later second century BCE, but this is a matter of debate, as we shall see), such verses gave an archaic tone to Nicander's poems. It certainly sounded familiar to the Greek readers of Nicander in antiquity since the *Iliad* and the *Odyssey* formed the backbone of ancient education and every educated Greek memorized them at an early age. Nevertheless, the use of such verses conveyed a sense of solemnity,

History of Toxicology and Environmental Health. DOI: http://dx.doi.org/10.1016/B978-0-12-800045-8.00006-X

majesty, and power—if not of inexorability and fatality—that strongly contrasted with the content of the two poems and the description of cases of poisoning and envenomation.

5.1 THE *THÊRIAKA*

The *Thêriaka* is about venomous animals. The title refers to wild animals (*thêr* in ancient Greek) and is an adjective in neuter, plural, functioning as a substantive meaning "the things about wild animals." The term *thêr* was normally used in classical Greek to refer to a wide variety of wild animals, from bears to wolves. Common to all of them was their possible noxiousness to humans. This notion justifies the use of the term *thêr* in the field of toxicology, but with the understanding that the possible harm arose from venom of the animals in question rather than the carnivorous qualities of creatures such as bears and wolves. Indeed, the toxicology of the time concerned itself with rather small animals such as scorpions, spiders, and insects.

The subjects of the *Thêriaka* are not limited to such obviously dangerous animals as those just mentioned (to which snakes of all kinds must be added). They also include other animals like shrews, lizards, and fishes. The common denominator in all such animals is the presence of both an anatomical structure that make it possible to inoculate a substance by transcutaneous injection, and a liquid that becomes harmful when injected into the human physiological system.

The anatomical structures functioning as needles may be the fangs of snakes, spiders, and shrews; the stings of scorpions, stingrays, and bees; or the acerate, needlelike dorsal fins of fishes. These structures allow for the inoculation of substances whose effects can range from irritant to lethal.

In this context, *Thêriaka* are the venomous animals identified as a group in the natural world. This group is not defined as a genus in terms of modern taxonomy, but rather by its anatomical structure, which allows for the inoculation of venom. In spite of this overarching definition, most of the *Thêriaka*—no less than 350 verses, or 40 percent of the whole work—is devoted to snakes.

The composition of the *Thêriaka* is clear. After the brief narration of two myths accounting for the creation of snakes and scorpions (verses 8–12 and 13–20, respectively), Nicander briefly mentions the activities of humans in the countryside that expose them to the risk of envenomation (verses 31–34). This is a pretext for him to introduce a tableau and to evoke country life in the manner of traditional Greek literature. Nicander then moves to the prevention of envenomation, mainly through fumigations with odoriferous substances that are supposed to repel snakes (verses 35–79) and body creams with the same objective (verses 80–114).

Once these preambles are finished, Nicander examines several cases of snake envenomation. Again, he opens this section with some tableaux, taking their substance from the description of the annual life cycle of snakes, their sloughing and breeding seasons (including the classical myth of female vipers killing their mates after coupling), and their supposed higher irritability (and hence the increased noxiousness of their venom) during scorching summer heat (verses 115–144). He then studies 15 snakes; for each one, he describes its habitat, body, and any other ethological characteristic, followed by a precise enumeration of the symptoms caused by envenomation (verses 145–492).

After this zoological-pathological section, Nicander devotes no less than 220 verses (493–713) to the treatment of the 15 cases of envenomation that he has just presented. He cites the ingredients for 23 remedies and explains how to prepare them. Strangely enough, he does not specify for which exact snake envenomation each remedy is used, whereas in the description of the symptoms following the different cases of envenomation, he makes clear the difference between hemolytic and neurotoxic venoms.

Demonstrating that his major focus is on snakes, Nicander analyzes all the other venomous animals in just 120 verses (715–836): spiders (715–768); scorpions (769–804); some insects (805–814); the shrew (815–816), which is supposed to be venomous but probably just propagates contagious diseases; lizards (817–821); and fishes (822–836).

The poem ends with a second section on therapeutics (verses 837–956). In no particular order, Nicander describes first and at great length a remedy made of 82 substances (verses 837–914). He then moves to emergency measures (verses 915–933), which include sucking the venom from the wound or applying leeches with the same purpose, applying cups and cauterization to aspire or burn the venom and close the wound, applying a tourniquet to prevent the diffusion of the venom in the cardiovascular system, and using irritant botanicals aimed at provoking hyperhemia to the same effect. The poems conclude with the description of a panacea made of 24 drugs.

5.2 THE *ALEXIPHARMAKA*

This second poem is substantially shorter than the *Thêriaka*, with just 630 verses. Its topic has not always been correctly understood. In the literature, it is not infrequent to find statements that the *Alexipharmaka* deals with the antidotes of venoms and poisons. Actually, the poem is devoted to poisons and poisoning and their treatment, and it represents the second part of the diptych that always constituted toxicology in antiquity, with the venoms on one side and the poisons on the other.

The meaning of the word *Alexipharmaka* is still unclear. It is manifestly composed of two elements, the second of which is *pharmakon*. In spite of its apparently obvious interpretation referring to a *remedy*, this term was used in antiquity to refer to both a remedy and a poison. Its exact meaning was defined by using a determinant (such as *esthlon* (salutary) or *kakon* (deadly) that helped clarify its fundamental ambiguity. This contradictory use indicates that the overarching meaning of *pharmakon* is neither "medicine" nor "poison," but rather "a substance introduced into the body (or applied to it) in order to provoke a modification." As for the first component of *Alexipharmaka*, *alex-*, it is of uncertain origin and meaning, although it clearly conveys the meaning of "treating" or "healing." The association of the two elements, *alex-* and *pharmakon*, may signify both the treatment (=*alex-*) of the deadly substances introduced into, or in contact with, the human body, or healing medicines (=*pharmakon*). Used as the title of this poem, it refers to the treatment of the funest effects of substances introduced into, or making contact with, the human body. This is all the more true because, if the *Alexipharmaka* is defined in that way, it completes the *Thêriaka* and constitutes the second half of the ancient toxicological discourse. In this way, the study of toxicology has two elements: venoms (injected by animals) and poisons (taken orally or through contact with the skin). The two parts make a coherent set of works on toxicology.

The structure of the *Alexipharmaka* is much more directly perceptible than that of the *Thêriaka*. It deals with 21 poisons from the three natural kingdoms (vegetable, mineral, and animal) and devotes a section to each of them, with three elements: the description of the solution containing the poison, that of the symptoms following its absorption *per os*, and finally, a list of remedies and their preparation.

5.3 THE NICANDREAN QUESTION

The Homeric style of the two poems is not limited to their form (i.e., each consists of 12 syllables); they both imply the epic mode, with its feeling of unicity, grandeur, and, at the same time, tragedy. In this view, the description of the symptoms that follow the envenomation or the poisoning is not strictly medical in nature—even though it uses medical terminology, sometimes specific and sometimes not. Rather, it is transformed into a grandiose epic battle between humans and death. The victims become heroes, fighting, with all their strength and energy, a desperate battle against a treacherous enemy, often hidden in the depth and the dark and attacking without a break in spite of the repeated administration of remedies.

Just as the Homeric epopee sometimes moves from the battlefield to the tents of the warriors on the plain of Troy and details the daily life of the soldiers, Nicander's narrative of the fight between humans and venoms/poisons is interrupted by descriptions of homes, with their cozy interiors, and of the quiet life of the countryside. For example, the variegated color of the skin of a snake is compared to a rug; the many leaves of a plant used for therapeutic purposes become a forest; and the inflammation of the body recalls the sun of summertime, together with the need for water and refreshment.

Delving deeper into these associations of ideas, the fight of humans against the destructive forces of venoms and poisons is equated to the primordial forces that shaped the cosmos; the narrative assumes a grandiose dimension with a desperate tone that inspires a feeling of tragedy.

This comparison of the report of clinical cases to the Homeric epopee with its multilayered interpretations, of which we have just highlighted some, poses the question of the exact nature of the *Thêriaka* and *Alexipharmaka* and of the identity of Nicander. Should the two poems be considered as medical works, or just literary fantasies on a medical theme? And what kind of background did their author have? Was he a physician with a perfect knowledge of toxicology, or a writer and a poet whose genius consisted of imbuing the toxicological discourse with an epic feeling? The toxicological knowledge—or the lack thereof—displayed in the two poems has rarely been taken into consideration in the polarized debate generated by these questions. Nor have the scanty elements known about Nicander's life been studied.

5.4 ANCIENT TOXICOLOGY

The knowledge of venoms and poisons in the ancient Greek world dates as far back as memory can go. In Greek mythology, Telegonus, son of Odysseus and the nymph Circe, accidentally killed his father with a spear topped with the venomous spine of a stingray. Although toxicology was not formalized as a discipline in its own right before the first century BCE/CE, it gradually developed into a coherent body of data organized according to a well-defined principle: the specificity of the action of the venoms and poisons, characterized by a selectivity for a determined physiological system in the human body. Such specificity required counteraction by means of equally specific therapies. As a result, when toxicology reached its peak sometime at the beginning of the Common Era, its discourse was organized according to this principle—that is, in a tripartite division: the description of the animals responsible for the envenomation or of the substances causing the poisoning for identification purposes and, on this basis, administration of the specific therapy; the description of their effect for the same reason, in case the lethal agent could not be seen or was no longer present; and the remedies.

The substance and the composition of the *Thêriaka* and *Alexipharmaka* do not demonstrate a full mastery of this principle or of the toxicological discourse. In the *Thêriaka*, the effects of hemolytic and neurotoxic venoms are distinguished very well and the text does not cause any confusion. However, no such distinction appears in the enumeration of the therapies that are grouped after the description of all the cases of envenomation. In the *Alexipharmaka*, the description of the substances and their effects instead is directly followed by a list of the therapies for such substance. Besides the differences in treatment between the *Thêriaka* and the *Alexipharmaka*, the lack of internal coherence in the *Thêriaka* does not support the hypothesis of Nicander as being a physician who was well informed and aware of the latest advances in toxicology. Rather, he seems to be a literate man who applied his art to create a paradoxical oeuvre.

5.5 VENOMS, POISONS, AND ART

Although his work is cited in some Greek and Latin literature, not much is known about Nicander. One of Nicander's works is dedicated to a king of Pergamon, usually identified as Attalus III, who reigned from 138 to 133 BCE. Attalus is reputed to have had a keen interest in toxicology, particularly in poisonous plants. He is credited with testing their effects via experiments on convicted criminals.

However unacceptable this might seem nowadays, it was not exceptional at the time, as other kings in that period did similar work. Besides the king of Macedonia, Antigonus II Gonatas (reigned 277–239 BCE), Antiochus III, king of Seleucia (reigned 222–187 BCE), and Ptolemy IV, king of Egypt (reigned 221–205 BCE), there was the king of Pontos, Mithridates VI Eupator (reigned 120–63 BCE), who distinguished himself by experiments of all kinds, including some that he performed on himself.

These kings give credibility to the activity of Attalus III of Pergamon and to the presence of a literate person at the royal court who devoted some of his works to the interest of his king. By writing these works in Homeric verses, the poet transformed (or maybe *transmuted* is a better word) the activities of his sovereign from a dubious activity into a literary expression of a drama of ancient daily life, particularly envenomation.

In perfect harmony with the artistic taste of his time and also in total continuity with the centuries-long Greek educational tradition, Nicander wrote the *Thêriaka* and *Alexipharmaka* in a Homeric way as a pathetic fight against death. His works are a graphical, almost visual representation of blood and gore, of violence and destruction, and of death and putrefied bodies. They echo the dramatic feeling of the Hellenistic time best concretized in the grandiloquent statuary of the Pergamon Altar. Simultaneously, the Homeric inspiration permeates the works with an epic sense of dignity as they compare the victims of poisons to the warriors whose heroic deeds shaped the Greek identity in history.

More than a diptych on toxicology, Nicander's *Thêriaka* and *Alexipharmaka* indicate the seductive power of venoms and poisons on the human imagination, however tragic this literary theme might be. As such, they have a place in the history of toxicology as an interesting source of information, however implicit and imperfect.

REFERENCE

[1] Gow AS, Schofield AF, editors. Nicander, the poems and poetical fragments. Edition with introduction, translation and notes. Cambridge: Cambridge University Press; 1953.

CHAPTER 6

Alexander the Great: A Questionable Death

Adrienne Mayor

On his way back to Greece after spectacular conquests from Persia to India, Alexander the Great (b. 356 BC) died in Babylon in the Palace of Nebuchadnezzar II (modern Iraq) on June 10 or 11, 323 BC. During one of many all-night drinking parties in Babylon, Alexander's companions had heard him cry out in pain, complaining of a "sudden, stabbing agony in the liver." The young conqueror of the known world was put to bed with severe abdominal pains and a very high fever. Over the next 12−14 days, his condition declined and he became gravely ill. The ancient sources report that Alexander suffered restlessness, weakness, extreme thirst, loss of consciousness, possible convulsions, and great pain. Partial paralysis set in—he was only able to move his eyes, head, and fingers with difficulty. He lost the ability to speak and fell into a deathlike state.

6.1 ALEXANDER'S LAST DAYS

Several ancient Greek and Roman historians described Alexander's last days. They had access to many contemporary texts that no longer survive, including a mysterious source called the "Royal Diaries" or "Journal" [1,2]. We know that five men close to Alexander wrote accounts of his death: Alexander's bodyguard and friend Ptolemy, his admiral Nearchus, his secretary Eumenes, his chamberlain Chares, and his military engineer Aristobulus. Unfortunately their memoirs are all lost except for fragmentary quotations preserved by later historians, including Diodorus Siculus (first century BC); Plutarch (about AD 100); Pliny and Quintus Curtius Rufus (both first century AD); Arrian, Pausanias, and Justin (second century AD); Aelian (about AD 200); and the so-called *History* or *Romance of Alexander* (dating to about AD 250; several manuscript versions exist).

According to Diodorus (17.117), at the last banquet he attended in Babylon, Alexander "drank much unmixed [strong] wine... and finally gulped down a huge beaker. Instantly he shrieked aloud as if struck by

History of Toxicology and Environmental Health. DOI: http://dx.doi.org/10.1016/B978-0-12-800045-8.00007-1

a violent blow." His attendants "conducted him to bed, and his physicians were summoned" but Alexander continued to suffer in great pain. Justin (12.13−15) adds more details: "Taking up a cup, he had drunk half of it when he suddenly uttered a groan, as if he had been pierced by a spear; he was carried half-conscious from the banquet. The torture was so excruciating that he called for a sword to put an end to it. The pain upon being touched by his attendants was if he were covered with wounds.... On the sixth day, he could no longer speak."

The historian Arrian (7.25−26) affirmed that Alexander was unable to speak near the end: "Lying speechless as his men filed by, he struggled to raise his head, and in his eyes there was a look of recognition for each individual as he passed." Justin (12.17) had also noted that Alexander was speechless but was able to move his hands: "Unable to speak, he took his ring from his finger, and gave it to Perdiccas [Alexander's trusted general]."

Alexander's biographer Plutarch (*Alexander* 75−77) denied the stabbing pain, describing only "a raging fever" marked by "violent thirst." Plutarch said "he drank a lot of wine, upon which he fell into delirium." Plutarch also described restlessness, loss of appetite, high fever, and inability to speak.

According to the third-century AD *Greek Alexander Romance* (3.30−31), which contains both historical facts and fantasy about Alexander's life and death, after his cupbearer Iolaus served him a beaker of wine late in the evening, Alexander began showing signs of malaise, getting up and pacing around the room. "He again sat down [and] with his hands trembling, complained that it was as if a heavy yoke were upon his neck. When he stood again to drink... he shouted with pain as if pierced in the liver with an arrow." The *Romance* continues: "[R]acked with pain," Alexander's condition deteriorated, and he "could not speak because his tongue was so swollen." He suffered convulsions, delirium, hallucinations, and bouts of unconsciousness. "Throughout the night the king would writhe and shake upon his bed, then he would become still. At other times he would ramble with meaningless words, appearing to speak with spirits in the bedchamber" [3].

About 13 days after falling ill at the banquet, Alexander was pronounced dead, on the afternoon of June 11, 323 BC, just before his 33rd birthday. His body was placed in a coffin in a storeroom. The Egyptian and Chaldean embalmers who arrived on June 16 noted that Alexander's body was strangely preserved, even in Babylon's hot climate (Plutarch *Alexander* 77; Curtius 9.19). This effect has been taken by modern historical detectives to indicate that some sort of poison may have preserved the corpse or that a profound coma was mistaken for death.

Many ancient Greek and Roman writers speculated on the true cause of Alexander's death, which remains an unsolved mystery. Several ancient historians reported that rumors of poisoning circulated soon after the untimely death of Alexander [4–6]. His closest friends suspected a legendary poison gathered from the Styx River waterfall near Nonacris in Arcadia (north central Peloponnese, Greece), a substance reputed to be so corrosive it could only be contained in the hoof of a horse. The Styx River was thought to be an entrance to the Underworld in classical antiquity and its waters were believed to be toxic.

The ancient historians were divided on whether Alexander died of natural causes or was murdered by poison. Justin (12.13–14) and Pliny (*Natural History* 30.53) accepted the poison conspiracy, as did Pseudo-Plutarch (*Lives of the Ten Orators* 56; *Moralia* 849 F). Pausanias (8.17.18), Arrian (7.27), and Curtius (10.10.14) were neutral. Plutarch (*Alexander* 75–77) was skeptical. Diodorus (17.117.5–118.1–2) was cautious, pointing out that after Alexander's bitter enemies, Antipater and Cassander, took over Alexander's empire, "many historians did not dare to write about the drug" or the plot. Moreover, he noted that Alexander's mother Olympias sought revenge on Cassander and others because she believed that they had poisoned her son (Diodorus 19.11.8). Olympias was then murdered by Cassander. Diodorus's intimations were more strongly expressed by Justin (12.13), who wrote, "The conspiracy... was suppressed by the power of Alexander's successors." In the Middle Ages and Renaissance, murder by poisoning was generally accepted as the cause of Alexander's death; Voltaire, among others, accepted the poisoning plot.

6.2 MODERN THEORIES OF NATURAL CAUSES

Many modern theories propose an array of natural causes for Alexander's slow death. These retrodiagnoses include alcohol poisoning from extremely heavy drinking, septicemia from infected old wounds that Alexander received on previous campaigns, pancreatitis, malaria, typhoid, West Nile fever, porphyria, schistosomiasis, accidentally harmful treatment by the royal physicians, or a combination of causes. In 2009, John Atkinson, Elsie Truter, and Etienne Truter produced a valuable summary and full bibliography of Alexander's last days, with the reported symptoms, a timeline based on the ancient sources, and an appendix of proposed causes of death and their merits and drawbacks [7].

Before falling ill in Babylon, Alexander had traveled across India, Pakistan, Iran, and Iraq. Hindu doctors accompanied his army in India and Pakistan; they provided Alexander with exotic natural medicinal plants, venoms, and minerals. Significantly, Alexander was known to have treated himself with unknown, powerful drugs—in one of these experiments he nearly died. One might speculate that some experimental self-treatment was the cause of his death [8].

It also may be significant that in the 2 weeks before his death Alexander had been sailing for 3 days in the Great Swamp of Babylonia, the marshy Tigris–Euphrates delta (Diodorus 17.116.5–7). This raises the possibility of mosquito-borne disease; many of the symptoms fit the ancient descriptions. West Nile fever has been suggested [9], but that is a recently evolved disease; perhaps an unknown precursor existed in Alexander's era. Malaria was first proposed by a French physician in 1878 and has been promoted by several recent historians [10–12]. Malaria is an attractive candidate, but the distinctive recurrent fever curve in malaria caused by the *Plasmodium* parasite was absent from the ancient reports. Typhoid has also been suggested [13,14]. A complication of typhoid is ascending paralysis, which could have caused Alexander to appear dead for several days before he died. But if any of these infectious diseases was the culprit, it seems likely that other people in Babylon would have been struck with similar symptoms. According to the detailed historical accounts, Alexander was the only one to fall ill, a fact that could point to poisoning.

6.3 MODERN THEORIES OF POISONING

Many modern arguments have been made for accidental or deliberate poisoning. In one theory, for example, Alexander's doctors treated him with a fatal dose of medicine in an attempt to counteract poisoning. Leo Schep, a toxicologist, considered what sort of drug might have been administered if Alexander was thought to have ingested poison; in 2009, he concluded that hellebore was the likely culprit [15]. In 2014, Schep's team suggested that if Alexander had been deliberately poisoned, it would have been by white hellebore (*Veratum album*) fermented into wine [16]. Arguments against hellebore include the following facts: hellebore is intensely bitter; there is no evidence for fermentation into wine in antiquity; and hellebore was notorious for causing violent gastrointestinal symptoms and even death in weak patients. Often prescribed as a purge in antiquity, hellebore had to be used very cautiously. The symptoms of hellebore poisoning were very well known generally and an overdose would have been recognized by Alexander's doctors and probably by his companions. The effects are unmistakable: hellebore induces explosive diarrhea and vomiting. Significantly, neither of these hallmark symptoms was mentioned in any of the ancient sources who described Alexander's death.

If Alexander was poisoned by his enemies, the agent may have been an easily available mineral or plant toxin. In 2004, Paul Doherty concluded that Alexander was poisoned with arsenic, which might have preserved the body from decomposition [17]. Strychnine was first suggested by R.D. Milnes [18], citing Theophrastus (*History of Plants* 9.11.5–6). In 2004, Graham Phillips [19] suggested an alkaloid plant such as belladonna (deadly nightshade), aconite (monkshood)—both easily available—or strychnine. Since Alexander did not suffer vomiting, which always accompanies alcohol, belladonna, arsenic, and aconite poisoning (as well as hellebore ingestion), Phillips concluded that the agent must have been strychnine (*Nux vomica*). Strychnine poisoning appears to match some of the symptoms: paroxysmal contractions of muscles followed by complete relaxation, skin very painful to touch, high fever, sweating, high blood pressure, intense thirst, and lockjaw. *Nux vomica* has a very bitter taste, however, making it difficult to hide in a drink. This plant would have had to come to Babylon from southern India, never reached by the Greeks. Moreover, poisoning by this and other plant toxins would have required repeated doses to cause Alexander's slow death, and this would increase the chances of the plot being discovered. It is also notable that Alexander, who was described as pathologically paranoid at this time, apparently did not himself suspect poisoning [10].

6.4 THE STYX RIVER POISON PLOT

Rumors of poisoning began to circulate among some of Alexander's companions soon after his death (Justin 12.14; Plutarch *Alexander* 77.1–3; Diodorus 17.118). Many people both in Babylon and in Macedon had the motives and the means. Suspicion fell on his enemy Antipater, the viceroy in Macedonia, and on Antipater's son Cassander, who had recently arrived in Babylon from Greece. Plutarch (*Alexander* 75–77) gives a detailed account of the alleged conspiracy and the special poison from the Styx, mentioned above. Some (such as Arrian 7.24–27; Plutarch *Alexander* 77; Pliny 30.53) claimed that it was Aristotle, Alexander's old friend and tutor, who had provided the Styx poison because he now feared his student. Aristotle was in Athens at the time of Alexander's death. He was said to resent the murder of his nephew by Alexander in 327 BC. Was Aristotle also suspected because he had written about Styx poison in a lost book of natural history? We know that Aristotle's fellow natural philosopher Theophrastus did write about Styx poison.

According to Arrian (7.24–27), "Antipater sent Alexander medicine which had been tampered with and he took it, with fatal results. Aristotle is supposed to have prepared this drug.... Antipater's son Cassander is said to have brought it [to Babylon]. Some accounts declare that he brought it in a mule's hoof, and that it was given to Alexander by Cassander's younger brother Iolaus, who was his cup-bearer.... [O]thers state that Medius, Iolaus' lover, had a hand in it.... [I]t was Medius who invited Alexander to the drinking-party [where Alexander] felt a sharp pain after draining the cup." The *Greek Alexander Romance* [3] maintained that the banquet was a conspiracy involving Antipater, Cassander, Iolaus, and others. Ingemar Düring [20] gathered and commented on the ancient evidence for Aristotle's involvement, and he suggested that the case was a common *topos* in public debates by later peripatetic philosophers. Plutarch (*Alexander* 75–77) identifies the authority for implicating Aristotle as Hagnothemis, who heard it from Antigonus, a trusted contemporary of Alexander. The Styx poison said to have been prepared by Aristotle was "deadly cold water from the rock cliff near Nonacris, gathered [or distilled] like a delicate dew [or exudation] and stored in an ass's hoof, for all other vessels were corrupted by its icy, penetrating corrosiveness."

According to the *Greek Alexander Romance*, Alexander was killed with a poison that destroyed bronze, glass, and clay, and had to be sealed in a lead jar inside an iron jar. When Alexander tried to induce vomiting to rid himself of the poison, Iolaus gave him a poisoned feather. A fourteenth-century illustrated manuscript of the *Greek Alexander Romance* contains miniature paintings depicting the poison being transported in a lead *pyxis* (lidded box) from Greece to Babylon, the poison passed to Iolaus the cupbearer, and Alexander drinking from a glass goblet. The motif of a feather coated with poison brings to mind the account of the poisoning of the Roman emperor Claudius, in Tacitus (*Annals* 12.56−58): when poisoned mushrooms prepared by the notorious poisoner Locusta failed to kill Claudius, the emperor called for a feather to induce vomiting but his doctor poisoned the feather. Some of Alexander's symptoms and the course of his illness seem to match ancient Greek myths about water from the Styx—for example, he lost his voice, like the Olympian gods who fell into a coma-like state after drinking from the Styx. This similarity of symptoms may have led his companions and others to assume (or to claim for propaganda purposes) that Styx poison was responsible. Such a sacred *pharmakon* or drug would cast an aura of divinity on Alexander. The notion that their great hero had succumbed to the fabled poison taken from the gods' sacred oath river would have carried symbolic resonance. Combined with ancient traditions associating the Styx with immortality, Alexander's friends could blame a mythic drug worthy of their "semidivine" leader.

The true cause of Alexander's untimely death more than 2300 years ago will probably never be solved with certainty. Even if Alexander *was* poisoned, the story of a strange "icy dew" gathered from the banks of the Styx waterfall, the dismal entrance to the Underworld, seems fantastic. Yet the descriptions of that poison and its source remained consistent in many different sources over many centuries. Although some of the historians and naturalists doubted the reality of a poison plot, not one ancient writer ever cast doubt on the existence of a deadly substance from the Styx River. Possible identifications of this toxin include calicheamicin, a deadly bacterium that thrives on limestone crust [21]. Scientific analysis might one day reveal the identity of a potentially deadly poison from the Styx. That would account for the river's nefarious reputation—but the demise of Alexander would still remain a mystery.

REFERENCES

[1] Badian E. A king's notebooks. Harv Stud Classic Philol 1968;72:183–204.

[2] Romm J. Ghost on the throne: the death of Alexander the Great and the war for crown and empire. New York, NY: Knopf; 2011.

[3] Stoneman, R. (trans.). The Greek Alexander Romance by Pseudo-Callisthenes. London: Penguin; 1991.

[4] Bosworth AB. The death of Alexander the Great: rumour and propaganda. Class Q 1971;21:112–36.

[5] Bosworth AB. Alexander's death: the poisoning rumors. In: Romm J, editor. The landmark Arrian: the campaigns of Alexander. New York, NY: Pantheon; 2010. p. 407–10.

[6] Lane Fox R. Alexander the Great. London: Penguin; 2004.

[7] Atkinson J, Truter E, Truter E. Alexander's last days: malaria and mind games? Acta Classica 2009;52 [January 1, n.p.] 23–46.

[8] Mayor A. The poison king: the life and legend of Mithradates, Rome's deadliest enemy. Princeton, NJ: Princeton University Press; 2010.

[9] Marr JS, Calisher CH. Alexander the Great and West Nile virus encephalitis. Emerg Infect Dis 2003;9:1599–603.

[10] Engels D. A note on Alexander's death. Class Philol 1978;73:224–8.

[11] Borza EN. Alexander's death: a medical analysis. In: Romm J, editor. The landmark Arrian: the campaigns of Alexander. New York, NY: Pantheon; 2010. p. 404–6.

[12] Thompson J. Disease, not conflict, ended the reign of Alexander the Great. Independent on Sunday 2011.

[13] Oldach D, Richard RE, Borza E, Benitez RM. A mysterious death. N Engl J Med 1998;338:1764–9.

[14] Cunha B. The death of Alexander the Great: malaria or typhoid fever? Infect Dis Clin North Am 2004:53–63.

[15] Schep L. The death of Alexander the Great: reconsidering poison. In: Wheatley P, Hannah R, editors. Alexander & his successors. Camas, WA: Regina Books; 2009. p. 227–36.

[16] Schep LJ, Slaughter RJ, Vale JA, Wheatley P. Was the death of Alexander the Great due to poisoning? Clin Toxicol 2014;52:72–7.

[17] Doherty P. The death of Alexander the Great: what—or who—really killed the young conqueror of the known world? New York, NY: Carroll and Graf; 2004.

[18] Milnes RD. Alexander the Great. New York, NY: Pegasus; 1968.

[19] Phillips G. Alexander the Great: murder in Babylon. London: HB Virgin Publishing; 2004.

[20] Düring I. Aristotle in the ancient biographical tradition. Göteborg: Almquist; 1957.

[21] Mayor A, Hayes A. The deadly Styx River of Greek myth: did poison from the Styx kill Alexander the Great? Poster, Toxicology History Room, XII International Congress of Toxicology, Barcelona, Spain; 2010.

CHAPTER 7

Harmful Botanicals

Alain Touwaide

7.1 CLASSICAL TOXICOLOGY

Medicinals of classical antiquity are generally considered the basis of the relatively recent development of Western drugs. In pharmacotherapy, a wide range of medicinals was drawn from the vast biodiversity of the Mediterranean environment. Significantly, the many plants used as *materia medica* for the preparation of remedies were also consumed daily as preventative formulations, of which the so-called Mediterranean diet—now redefined as the "Greek diet"—is the modern avatar.

Unsurprisingly, the knowledge and judicious use of natural resources for the management of health, be it curative or preventative, went together with awareness of the potential dangers (from mind alteration to death) of some botanicals. This resulted in the development of methods aimed at counteracting their effects.

7.2 SOURCES AND DATA

Knowledge of potentially harmful botanicals is evident in the written legacy of ancient Greece and mythological references are ubiquitous in this literature. The magician, Circe, daughter of the Sun and of the Oceanid Perse, i.e., the elements that shaped the cosmos, is said to have used botanicals to convert the companions of Odysseus into swine (*Odyssey*, 10.475–541).

In this chapter, knowledge of harmful botanicals in classical antiquity is drawn from the ancient medical and scientific literature. Although information on natural toxic substances can be found in the most ancient body of Greek medical literature currently preserved [namely, the series of over 60 treatises ascribed to Hippocrates (between

History of Toxicology and Environmental Health. DOI: http://dx.doi.org/10.1016/B978-0-12-800045-8.00008-3

375 and 350 BCE) and forming what is called the *Hippocratic Collection*], it is not specific and does not communicate an exact understanding of the ancient knowledge about toxic plants. Nevertheless, it is useful for chronological purposes and for a reconstruction of the development of what can be called *classical toxicology*—in other words, a body of data on a determined object, organized according to specific parameters, aiming at a relevant objective, and forming, if not a discipline, at least a specialty that is explicitly recognized as such. The best source about classical toxicology defined in this way is a pair of treatises ascribed to Dioscorides (dating from the first century CE), the author of *De materia medica,* the most famous encyclopedia of *materia medica* of antiquity. One of these two documents deals with poisons of all kinds (*De venenis*), and the other covers animal venoms (*De venenosis animalibus*).

Though certainly not written by Dioscorides himself, these two treatises reflect the development in the knowledge of poisons and venoms of the period (during the first century CE). At any rate, they had a diffusion that was almost as exceptional as that of *De Materia Medica*, as they provided the basis of virtually all the subsequent written works on toxicological matters—from Galen (129–c.216 CE) himself, however eager he was to always reformulate the legacy of previous generations and to reinterpret and integrate it into his own thinking; to such typical Byzantine medical encyclopedists as Theophanes Chrysobalantes in the tenth century; Oribasius in the fourth century; Aetius and Alexander of Tralles in the sixth century; and Paul of Egina, the last physician of Alexandria, in the seventh century. Arabic and medieval physicians also used the pseudo-Dioscoridean treatises as a source of the treatment of toxicology in their medical works, be they all-encompassing encyclopedias or shorter treatises specifically devoted to toxicology. The two treatises ascribed to Dioscorides thus appear to have formed the backbone of most premodern knowledge of natural harmful substances, be they botanicals, minerals, or animals. Such substances included the venoms injected by snakes, scorpions, fishes, and insects, and the bites of rabid dogs. Such continuity in the transmission and use of the treatises ascribed to Dioscorides does not preclude the fact that original works developed over time, including theoretical reflections on the concept of poison itself. The fact is that the body of data contained in these works provided the basic information for almost all material on the topic for approximately 15 centuries, even though this set of data may have been reformulated, expanded, or revised.

Of the two treatises, the most relevant here is the one entitled *On Deleterious Substances and Their Prevention* (= *De venenis*). It contains 34 chapters totaling over 600 lines and 5000 words. After a first long chapter dealing with general considerations, each of the subsequent 33 chapters is devoted to one harmful natural substance: 10 animals (plus the honey produced by bees that have taken the pollen of a toxic plant), 16 plants, and 5 minerals. The common denominator of all these substances (regardless of the natural kingdom to which they pertain) is that they are taken orally, as opposed to those in the twin treatise *De venenosis animalibus*, incorrectly ascribed to Dioscorides, in which all substances (exclusively animal in nature) are injected into the body or come into contact with the skin.

In the treatise *De venenis*, all the chapters (whatever the nature of the harmful substance) are built from a template made of three parts: (1) the organoleptic description of the substance, (2) the description of the clinical signs following its absorption, and (3) the therapies aimed at counteracting its effects. The parts are not dealt with in the same way or with the same degree of detail in each chapter. As an example of this template, here is the discussion of hemlock (Chapter 11):

> **On hemlock.** Hemlock taken in a draught may cause scotomy (dizziness and dimness of sight), possibly leading to blindness, as well as hiccups, impaired intellectual capacity, and cold extremities. It may ultimately result in convulsions and suffocation due to choking.
>
> At the beginning, we will eliminate it [=hemlock] as in any other case, that is, by [having the patients] vomiting. Further on, using evacuation, we will eliminate the portion [of hemlock] that has arrived into the intestines. Then, we will use wine as the best remedy, giving it with intervals during which we will give donkey milk or absinth with pepper and wine; castorium and rue with wine; cardamon or storax or pepper with nettle seeds and wine; or laurel leaves, silphium and its juice with oil and sweet wine; and also sweet wine itself abundantly administered will help pretty much.

The plants whose harmful effects are analyzed are listed in the table on the next page in alphabetical order according to their current English names when available. The table provides the number of the chapter devoted to each one in the treatise *De venenis*, together with its Linnaean binomial designation.

English Name	Number	Scientific Identification	Dioscorides	Notes
Buttercup	14	*Ranunculus sardous* Crantz	2.175	[1, pp. 690–2]
Coriander	9	*Coriandrum sativum* L.	3.63	[2], pp. 39–41. The toxicity attributed to coriander in antiquity (that is, mind-altering) probably results from contamination or the ingestion of high doses of the plant [3]
Doruknion	6	*Convolvulus oleaefolius* Desr.	4.74	[4, p. 406]
Efemeron	5	*Colchicum autumnale* L.	4.83	[1, pp. 693–702]
Farikon	19	N/A	N/A	Not identified; probably a Solanacea.
Fleawort	10	*Plantago psyllium* L.	4.69	[4, p. 245]
Hemlock	11	*Conium maculatum* L.	4.78	[1, pp. 796–9]
Henbane	15	*Hyoscyamus* spp.	4.68	[1, pp. 776–83]
Honey from Heraklea	8	Honey from bees having absorbed the pollen of *Rhododendrum* spp.	2.82	[1, pp. 870–2]
Horned poppy	18	*Glaucium flavum* L.	4.65	[4, pp. 275–6]
Mandrake	16	*Mandragora autumnalis* L. or *M. officinalis* L.	4.75	[1, pp. 779–80]
Mushrooms	23	Multiple species	4.82	For gastroenteritis-producing species [1, pp. 290–3]
Pine thistle	21	*Atractylis gummifera* L.	3.8	[1, pp. 514–16]
Poppy juice	17	*Papaver somniferum* L.	4.64	[4, p. 225]
Toxikon	20	N/A	N/A	Not identified; supposed to be the plant whose juice was smeared on arrows (hence its name, as *toxon* means arrow)
White hellebore	13	*Veratrum album* L.	4.148	[1, pp. 815–18]
Wolfsbane	7	*Aconitum napellus* L.	4.77	[1, pp. 736–42]
Yew	12	*Taxus baccata* L.	4.79	[1, pp. 899–901]

7.3 ANALYSIS

In antiquity, the aim of the medical specialty dealing with harmful substances (including botanicals) was to cure the victim of poisoning, be it the result of a mistake or a criminal action. The therapeutic strategy of the time was guided by the principle that each toxic substance has a specific, typical action. Hence, the therapy needed to counteract such action in an equally specific way, with appropriate therapeutic means according to a principle explicitly mentioned in the treatise ascribed to Dioscorides (see 8.12–13). This general principle, which clearly results from a long-term examination of the differentiated effects of the range of botanicals above (and probably of many others, but not necessarily those leading to life-threatening conditions), defined the therapeutic strategy of physicians in their treatment of cases. It also defined the content and structure of the chapters devoted to each substance and the general structure—that is, the sequence of the chapters—of the treatise ascribed to Dioscorides and those which followed it. In addition, it reproduced its information from antiquity to the dawn of modern science.

With regard to the chapters devoted to each substance, each is divided into three parts in most cases, as I have mentioned. The first two parts (that is, the organoleptic description of the poisonous substances and the description of their effects, possibly including some pathological mechanism, supposed or real) aim to identify the poison in order to apply the appropriate therapy. The first one relies on the assumption that the draft through which the noxious substance has been administered is still available. The examination of the organoleptic qualities of a substance—which includes everything but tasting it, which would harm the physician— should lead to the substance's identification, after which a specific therapy can be directly administered. If the causal agent is no longer available (which may be the case, particularly with criminal poisoning), it should be eliminated from the body of the patient via vomiting. If this can be done soon after the absorption of the lethal drink, the causal agent can be identified again by its organoleptic properties.

If the poisoning cup is not available or vomiting cannot be quickly provoked, identification of the harmful substance should be made through the disturbances that it causes to the victims. This is the rationale of the clinical description of the symptoms following the absorption of the toxins. These symptomatologies are relatively short, as they aim to stress the major characteristics of the toxic action of each substance in order to reach a rapid and precise diagnosis. They clearly rely on the repeated observation of multiple clinical cases, the recording of all the signs following the absorption of harmful substances by humans, and the isolation of the most common signs, further expressed in an essential way, as an abstract concept. Such abstraction is certainly not the result of the work of a determined individual (such as, for example, the author of the treatise ascribed to Dioscorides). Actually, it is the product of years, if not centuries, of observations, possibly first transmitted in an unorganized way by means of oral tradition and popular knowledge and then transferred the world of physicians and written down, codified, and standardized into proper technical language. During the last phase of its codification, such knowledge may have continued to be refined, clarified, and made more accurate and complete (and, consequently, also more efficient), finally taking the form that it has in the treatise attributed to Dioscorides.

It was the role of the practitioner to interpret the symptoms of the patient he was treating and to repeat the exercise of abstraction of his predecessors. This was done for the purpose of extracting from an actual case its most salient pathological signs, to compare them with the clinical descriptions in the literature (that is, a treatise like the one attributed to Dioscorides), and to ascertain that the case he was treating corresponded to one in the literature. On this basis, he had to apply the therapy specifically prescribed for this case.

In this diagnostic process, physicians probably proceeded in a gradual way, step by step. In the treatise *On Poisons*, we note that the several harmful substances are grouped not by natural kingdom (as one might expect), but by major categories of effects. Using the descriptions from the ancient text—that is, the symptoms attributed to each toxin, with no attempt to identify their causal mechanisms—there are six major groups of actions. For each one, the substances that provoke it are in parentheses, and, for each substance, the number of the chapter is given in squared brackets:

- Lesions of the digestive system (*doruknion* [6], *efemeron* [5], honey from Heraclea [8], wolfsbane [7])
- Dramatic reduction of body temperature (fleawort [10], hemlock [11], white hellebore [13], yew [12])
- Troubles of the Mind (buttercup [14], coriander [9], henbane [15], mandrake [16])

- Deep sleep and loss of consciousness (horned poppy [18], poppy [17])
- Impaired mobility and paralysis (*farikon* [19])
- Harsh irritation of the mouth; swelling and, consequently, obstruction of the alimentary tract (mushrooms [23], pine thistle [21], *toxikon* [20])

The first phase in the diagnostic process consisted of identifying one of these major actions. As is shown by the chapter numbers, all substances with a similar or identical action were grouped together.

Once a major action had been identified, the physician needed to distinguish more precisely the agent within the group. The symptoms attributed to each substance are listed with increased differentiation, proceeding almost by binary choices. This process can be summarized as follows, assuming that we have a group of three substances and that symptom A is the one that characterizes the whole group:

- If only symptom A is present, then the substance is labeled 1.
- If symptom A is accompanied by symptom B, then the substance is labeled 2.
- If symptom B is absent, if it was replaced by symptom C, or if it is present and accompanied by symptom C, then the substance is labeled 3.

This means that the method for the proper identification of a specific toxin was differential, consisting of grouping together all the substances with a similar or identical action, comparing their symptoms, and finally identifying exclusive symptoms, leading to a precise identification of the poison. Therapy was administered on that basis.

As a consequence of the lack of understanding of the pathological mechanisms, therapies were limited to treating the symptoms rather than the causes, something that drastically reduced their efficacy in spite of their sheer number and great variety. Nevertheless, in the case of subacute intoxication, it is highly probable that therapies may have compensated for the actions of the toxic agents during the crisis phase, allowing the patients to survive.

Regarding the period when this system was created, we noticed that it cannot be traced in any form to the vast collections of treatises ascribed to Hippocrates, which span between the fifth century BCE and the second century CE. It can be recognized, though only partially, in the *De materia medica* of Dioscorides (first century CE), since the work, dealing with *materia medica* specifically, does not include considerations of the pathologies that may have been generated by botanicals. However, the grouping of *materia medica* by action (and, in our specific case, by pathological action) is present in the work. In the second and early third centuries, this system was no longer present as such in the treatise *De venenis*, as the substances were grouped by natural kingdoms and each one is listed in alphabetical order according to the Greek name. All the information linked with the grouping, therefore, is lost. Nevertheless, the general principle of the system that we have reconstructed through the pseudo-Dioscoridean *De venenis* (that is, the necessity of a specific treatment based on the identification of relevant symptoms), can be found in a scattered form in Galen's many works. It thus seems that the development of a toxicological method with a theoretical system accounting for the written works that have come to us dates back to the first century CE, and probably somewhat earlier, because the achievements of the first century CE may have caused the disappearances of their predecessors.

Extant documentation includes fragments or traces of works on toxicological matters by physicians of the Alexandrian school during the third century BCE. Nevertheless, judging from the scanty remains, such works seem to have been limited to anatomo-pathological analysis, rather than to a theorization about a body of facts observed by experience. Furthermore, during the second century BCE, the work of Nicander, though it demonstrates good knowledge of the activity of poisons, neither includes a classification nor, on this basis, elements of differential diagnosis as in the pseudo-Dioscoridean treatise *De venenis*. It is reasonable to speculate that the system of toxicology presented above and defined here as classical toxicology dates back to the period between the fading of the medical school of Alexandria and the zenith of Greek medicine in the first century of the Roman Empire—that is to say, between the first century BCE and the end of the first century CE.

7.4 CONCLUSION

The system that we describe here is not explicitly presented in the pseudo-Dioscoridean treatise *De venenis* or in any of its subsequent heirs. Nevertheless, both the grouping of the substances and the presentation of the symptoms of each substance within the groups are clear enough to allow such a reconstruction. Although the pathological mechanisms generating the effects taken into consideration in order to identify the causal agents were not perceived, the system was efficient—at least for the identification of harmful botanicals, if not for the treatment of the effects following their absorption by humans. This probably accounts for the exceptional fortuna of the body of knowledge created in antiquity.

REFERENCES

[1] Barceloux DG. Medical toxicology of natural substances. Foods, fungi, medicinal herbs, plants and venomous animals. Hoboken, NJ: Wiley; 2008.

[2] Frohne D, Pfänder HJ. Poisonous plants. 2nd edition. A handbook for doctors, pharmacists, toxicologists, biologists and veterinarians. Portland, OR: Timber Press; 2004.

[3] Leclerc H. Précis de phytothérapie. Essais de thérapeutique par les plantes françaises[4]. Paris: Masson; 1954.

[4] van Wyk B-E, Wink M. Medicinal plants of the world. An illustrated scientific guide to important medicinal plants and their uses. Portland, OR: Timber Press; 2004.

CHAPTER 8

The Case Against Socrates and His Execution

Okan Arihan, Seda Karaoz Arihan and Alain Touwaide

8.1 INTRODUCTION

The Greek philosopher Socrates (469–399 BC) is famous in the history of Western thinking for constantly asking questions and pressing his interlocutors in inquisitive dialogues that were immortalized by his disciple Plato (428/7–348/7 BC). In 399 BC, he was sentenced to death by the senate of Athens because he supposedly corrupted the Athenian youth and did not respect the gods.

According to historiographical tradition, Socrates was given a poisonous draught whose ingredients have been discussed by modern authors. Whereas it has been traditionally considered to be hemlock, some thought it was hemlock and opium, and others believed it to have been other ingredients.

Hemlock (*kôneion* in ancient Greek) is now identified as *Conium maculatum* L. It is among the most toxic plants of the *Apiaceae* family and is commonly found in the flora of the Mediterranean region and Greece [1]. Although its toxicity had been known since antiquity, it was not studied scientifically until 1760, when it was discussed by the Austrian physician Anton von Stoerck (1731–1803). His [2] work on the subject was first published in Latin under the title *Libellus, quo demonstratur: cicutam non solum usu interno tutissime exhiberi, sed et esse simul remedium valde utile in multis morbis, qui hucusque curatu impossibiles dicebantur* and translated the same year into English as *An essay on the medicinal nature of hemlock: in which its extraordinary virtue and efficacy, as well internally as externally used, in the cure of cancers... are demonstrated.*

The main biologically active component of hemlock is the alkaloid coniine, which was isolated in 1827 by the German chemist August Louis Giseke [3]. Its structure was later clarified by August Wilhelm Hoffmann (1818–1892) [4]. Hemlock has frequently been cited in literature on poisonings since antiquity; studies of the bioactivity and pharmacological properties of coniine were initiated as early as 1898 [5].

History of Toxicology and Environmental Health. DOI: http://dx.doi.org/10.1016/B978-0-12-800045-8.00009-5

The mechanism of the action of coniine was clarified more recently. Its action on the nervous system is by the nicotinic acetylcholine receptors [6]. It stimulates the ganglions, and this stimulation is followed by a ganglionic blockade; finally, asphyxia occurs after the blockage of the phrenic nerves, which are responsible for breathing [7].

Coniine was once a popular molecule in medical research. However, the antinociceptive properties of coniine were not studied until 2009 [8].

8.2 HISTORICAL LITERATURE

Although much literature has been devoted to Socrates' last days, the textual evidence brought to light so far has been scanty.

To compensate for this lacuna, we have identified the following texts as sources of primary information for the analysis of Socrates' death (we list them in alphabetical order according to each ancient author's name):

- Aelian (second/third century AD) [9], author of the vast collection of data on animals entitled *Natura animalium* (*On the characteristics of animals*) [10].
- Andocides (440—after 392/1 BC) [11], Attic orator, author of discourses including *On the peace with Sparta* [12].
- Aristophanes (d. in the 380s BC) [13], author of comedies, among which the *Ranae* (*Frogs*) [14].
- The so-called *Corpus Hippocraticum* [15], that is, a series of 60 + treatises produced between the late fifth century BC and the second century AD and attributed to Hippocrates (460—between 375 and 351 BC) [16].
- Diodorus of Sicily (first century BC) [17], a historian who wrote a *Bibliothêkê* (Library) in 40 books covering the whole history of the world from its beginning up to the middle of the first century BC [18].
- Diogenes Laertius (mid-third century AD) [19] composed a series of biographies of philosophers (*Vitae philosophorum—Lives of the Philosophers*), including Socrates [20].
- Dioscorides (first century AD) [21], compiler of *De materia medica*, the largest encyclopedia of antiquity on the natural substances (of plant, animal, and mineral origin) used for the preparation of medicines [22,23].

- The treatise *On poison* attributed to Dioscorides [24], although probably not written by him, and added to *De materia medica* at a certain point in time, at any rate before the ninth century AD [25,26].
- Galen of Pergamum (AD 129—after 216 [?]) [27] abundantly wrote on all medical topics. Of interest here are three of his treatises:
  - *De simplicium medicamentorum temperamentis ac facultatibus* (*On the mixtures and properties of simple medicines*) [28]
  - *De morborum causis* (*On the causes of diseases*) [29,30]
  - *De alimentorum facultatibus* (*On the properties of food*) [29,30]
- Nicander of Colophon (third/second century BC) [31], author of the most ancient Greek works currently known on poisons and venoms [32].
- Plato (428/7—348/7 BC) [33], the disciple of Socrates and the author of several philosophical dialogues, among which *Euthyphron*, *Crito*, and *Phaedo* are of particular interest here [34,35].
- Pliny (AD 23/4—79) [36], a contemporary of Dioscorides (above) and the author of the *Historia Naturalis* (*Natural History*), which is an all-encompassing encyclopedia of the natural historical knowledge of his time [37].
- Plutarch of Chaeronea (ca. AD 45 and before AD 125) [38]. A prolific writer, he compiled a set of biographies in which he compared Greeks and Romans who had an important role in history, the so-called *Vitae parallelae* (*Parallel Lives*) [39].
- Seneca (d. AD 65) [40], a Roman philosopher who wrote a series of moral essays (*Moralia*) on different topics such as *De providentia* [41] and exchanging *Letters* (*Epistulae*) with his friend Lucilius in which he discussed all manners of moral topics [42].
- Theophrastus (371/0—287/6 BC), a disciple of Aristotle (384—322 BC) [43] and the author of *Historia plantarum* (*Inquiry into Plants*) [44], considered to be the foundational work of botany.
- Xenophon of Athens (ca. 430—354 BC) [45], the author, among others, of the *Hellenica* (or *Greek History*) [46].

On the basis of these sources, we have collected the following data:

a. We have one main account of Socrates' death by a contemporary, based on a personal autoptic participation in the event, in the *Phaedo* (117a—118) by Plato.

b. The term used by Plato to identify the substance absorbed by Socrates is generic: *poison* (*farmakon* in ancient Greek). This is also the case in Seneca's *Letter to Lucilius* (*Letter* 104: *venenum*). In his essay *On Providence*, Seneca uses the generic term *potio* (*draught*) (3.12), which does not contain any notion of toxicity. Nevertheless, Diodorus of Sicily and Diogenes Laertius both explicitly mention hemlock (*kôneion* in classical Greek) (Diodorus, 14.37.7; Diogenes, 2.5 [=*Life of Socrates*], §35).

c. Passages in ancient nonscientific literature confirm that hemlock was used in Athens as a lethal agent during Socrates' lifetime and in the following century (passages below are listed in the chronological order of the cases they report):

- 405 BC: Aristophanes, in the *Frogs*, mentions hemlock as the quickest way to commit suicide (124). Also, he says that many ladies took hemlock because they could not stand "the shame and sin" of certain situations (1051).
- 404 BC: Xenophon, in the *Greek History*, 2.3.56, reports a death due to hemlock.
- 404/3 BC: Andocides, in *On the peace with Sparta*, 20, mentions that, during the oligarchy of the Thirty (that is, during the year 404/3 BC), "many citizens [died] by the hemlock-cup."
- Between 399 and 387: Plato mentions hemlock in *Lysis* (219e), in the scene where he discusses a son and his father, with the son having drunk hemlock and the father doing all he can to save him. This dialogue was written after Socrates' death (399) and before Plato's first trip to Sicily in 387 BC.
- 318 BC: Diodorus of Sicily (18.64−67) and Plutarch (Life of Phocion 31−37) reports that the Athenian orator, politician, and general Phocion (402/1−318 BC) was sentenced to death and forced to ingest hemlock.

d. The action of the poison ingested by Socrates is described as follows by Plato (*Phaedo* 117b−e):

the man ... was to administer the poison, which he brought with him in a cup ready for use. And when Socrates saw him, he said: "Well, my good man, you know about these things: what must I do?" "Nothing," he replied, "except drink the poison and walk about till your legs feel heavy and the poison will take effect of itself." ... He walked about and, when he said his legs were heavy, lay down on his back, for such was the advice of the attendant. The man who had administered the poison laid his hands on him and after a while examined his feet and legs, then pinched his foot hard and asked if he felt it.

He said "No"; Then after that, his thighs; and passing upwards in this way he showed us that he was cold and rigid. And again he touched him and said that when it reached his heart, he would be gone. The chill had now reached the region about the groin, and uncovering his face, which had been covered, he said—and these were his last words—"Crito, we owe a cock to Aesculapius. Pay it and do not neglect it." "That," said Crito, "shall be done; but see if you have anything else to say." To this question he made no reply, but after awhile he moved; the attendant uncovered him; his eyes were fixed.

8.3 HEMLOCK IN ANCIENT SCIENTIFIC LITERATURE

Botanical information on hemlock can be found in the following works (in chronological order; to find relevant information we needed to expand the chronological frame, using works posterior to Socrates' time);

- Theophrastus, *Inquiry into plants*
- Dioscorides, *De materia medica*
- Pliny, *Natural History*

In this body of literature, hemlock is described as follows:

- Theophrastus, *Inquiry into plants*:
  - "Next of the woods themselves and of stems generally some are fleshy, as in... hemlock..." (1.5.3).
  - "Of the others some to a certain extent resemble ferula, that is, in having a hollow stem; for instance... hemlock..." (6.29).
  - "Mountain-celery (parsley) exhibits even greater differences; its leaf is like that of hemlock..." (7.6.4).
  - "Hemlock is best about Susa and in the coldest spots. Most of these plants (that is, the medicinal plants) occur also in Laconia, for this too is a land rich in medicinal plants" (9.15.8).
- Dioscorides, *De materia medica*, 4.78. The text reads as follows:
  - "Hemlock: it sends up a large stem, knotty like fennel, leaves look like those of giant fennel, but narrower and oppressive in scent; at the top it has side-shoots and umbels of whitish flowers; it has seeds like of anise but whiter, and a root that is hollow and not deep."
- Pliny, *Natural History*:
  - "... the stem is smooth, and jointed like a reed, of a dark colour, often more than two cubits high, and branchy at the top; the leaves resemble those of coriander, but are more tender, and of a strong smell; the seed is coarser than that of anise, the root hollow and of no use..." (25.151).

Extant medico-pharmaceutical literature contemporary to Socrates does not contain much relevant information on the action of hemlock on human physiology. Consequently, we expanded the chronological frame by including in our inquiry works of subsequent periods up to the second and early third century AD. Relevant data are the following (in chronological order of the works):

- The *Corpus Hippocraticum*:
  - The fruit of hemlock is ground with wine for a plaster to treat fistulae (6.458.16).
  - Hemlock is administered as a draught with water as an emmenagogue after childbirth (7.356.13).
  - Administration of a mixture of sulfur, asphalt, hemlock, or myrrh with honey as an anal injection to treat *hysteria* (8.278.9).
  - Fumigation with hemlock, or myrrh or incense, together with perfume, to treat red discharges (8.378.10).
  - Application of a mixture made of nightshade and hemlock previously boiled together to treat red discharges (8.380.11).
  - Fumigation with hemlock leaves to treat a female sterility (8.432.18).
- Theophrastus, *Inquiry into plants*:
  - "... in hemlock the juice is stronger and it causes an easier and speedier death even when administered in a quite small pill; and it is also more effective..." (9.8.3).
- Nicander, *Alexipharmaka*:
  - "Take note too of the noxious draught which is hemlock, for this drink assuredly looses disaster upon the head bringing the darkness of night: the eyes roll, and men roam the streets with tottering steps and crawling upon their hands; a terrible choking blocks the lower throat and the narrow passage of the windpipe; the extremities grow cold; and in the limbs the stout arteries are contracted; for a short while the victim draws breath like one swooning, and his spirit beholds Hades." (186–194).
- Dioscorides, *De materia medica*:
  - "This one, too, belongs to the plants that are deadly, killing by chilling through and through." (4.78).
- Pliny, *Natural History*:
  - "Hemlock too is poisonous, a plant with a bad name because the Athenians made it their instrument of capital punishment, but its

uses for many purposes must not be passed by. It has a poisonous seed, but the stem is eaten by many both as a salad and when cooked in a saucepan.... The seed and leaves have chilling quality, and it is this that causes death; the body begins to grow cold at the extremities..." (25.150).

- Seneca, *On Providence*:
  - "... his blood grew cold, and, as the chill spread, gradually beating of his pulses stopped..." (3.12).
- Galen:
  - *On the mixtures and properties of simple medicines*:
    - "Everybody knows that hemlock is of the outmost cooling property." (7.10.67).
  - *On the causes of diseases*:
    - "Among the cooling drugs are... hemlock, the last of which is lethal because of its violent chilling action. We designate the blockage as the third and worst cause of cooling diseases, since it engenders torpor, lethargy and apoplexy." (7.13.17-14.6).
- Aelian, *On the characteristics of animals*:
  - "... if a man drinks hemlock, he dies from the congealing and chilling of his blood..." (4.23).
- Pseudo-Dioscorides, *On poisons*:
  - "In a draught, hemlock provokes a loss of vision at such point to be blind, gasping, a loss of consciousness and cold in the extremities; at the end, the victims gasp as they are asphyxied because breath stops." (11).

Representations of hemlock can be found in several Byzantine manuscripts containing the Greek text of Dioscorides, *De materia medica*. We have considered only the most ancient ones (cited below in chronological order), since the most recent are copies of one or another of them:

- Vienna, National Library of Austria, *medicus graecus* 1 (sixth cent.), f. 187 verso.
- Paris, National Library of France, *graecus* 2179 (ninth cent.), f. 106 recto.
- New York, Pierpont Morgan Library, M 652 (tenth cent.), 76 recto.
- Mt Athos, Megistis Lavras, Ω 75 (11th cent.), f. 61 recto.

No particularly significant information on hemlock and its uses was found in nontechnical literature beyond those mentioned above, under 1. c), apart from the belief that some animal species were immune to the effect of hemlock:

- Starlings, according to Galen (On *properties of food* 6.567.14)
- Swans, according to Aelian (3.7)
- Hogs, according to the same (4.23)

A particular point is the question of the preparation of hemlock for its medicinal use, on which we have some information coming from technical and nontechnical literature (in chronological order according to author).

- Theophrastus, in the *Inquiry into Plants* (9.16.8–9), details the way hemlock has to be prepared to be used as a lethal agent:
  "Thrasyas of Mantinea has discovered, as he said, a poison which produces an easy and painless end; he used the juices of hemlock, poppy, and other such herbs, so compounded as to make a dose of conveniently small size... he used to gather his hemlock, not just anywhere, but at Susa or some other cold and shady spot... he also used to compound many other poisons, using many ingredients... the people of Kos formerly did not use hemlock in the way described, but just shredded it up for use, as did other people; but now they first strip off the outside and take off the husk, since this is what causes the difficulty, as it is not easily assimilated; they then bruise it in the mortar, and, after putting it through a fine sieve, sprinkle it on water and so drink it; and then death is made swift and easy."
- Seneca, in his essay *On Providence* (3.12), specified that the draught taken by Socrates had been *mixed publicly* (*publice mixtam*), a piece of information implying that there were several ingredients. However, he did not detail the ingredients.
- In the *Life of Phocio* by Plutarch, we read the following (36.2):
  - "... seeing the executioner bruising the hemlock..."

The plant identified in ancient Greek by means of the word *kôneion* is unanimously identified by the post-Linnean authors of botanico-historical works as *Conium maculatum* L. from the *Florae Graecae Prodromus* (1806–1813) by the Englishman John Sibthorp (1756–1798) [47] to, recently, Suzanne Amigues [48].

The post-Linnean flora of Greece confirm that hemlock (=*Conium maculatum* L.) is present in the area corresponding to modern Greece. According to Sibthorp, in the *Florae Graecae Prodromus* (1806–1813) [47], it was common in the area of Athens. According to Edmond Boissier (1872), author of a *Flora orientalis*, it can be found in all of Europe except Lapponia, North Africa, Abyssinia, and Syria. According to his *Conspectus Florae Graecae*, de Halacsy found it in 1901 [49] in Attica and the region of Athens. Boissier, in the *Supplementum* of his *Flora* published in 1908, added the Attica [50]. More recently, Hegi described it in the *Flora of Mittel-Europa* as omnipresent in Europe, Asia, and North Africa, while the *Flora Europaea* [51] describes it as typical of almost all Europe except the extreme north [52].

A comparison of ancient textual data, representations in manuscripts, dry specimens from herbaria, and descriptions in modern flora confirms the following:

• The ancient Greek word *kôneion* corresponds to the taxon currently identified as *Conium maculatum* L.
• The plant grows in the area that comprised the ancient Greek world and probably grew there in antiquity.

In modern literature, the most relevant analysis from our viewpoint here is provided by the German toxicologist Louis Lewin (1850–1929) [53]. Capitalizing on the work of his predecessors, he listed and paraphrased in his magisterial work *Die Gifte in der Weltgeschichte* (*Poisons in World History*) (1920) the several historical cases of death provoked by means of hemlock in ancient Greece, specifically in Athens. After he commented on Theophrastus' passage, cited above, about the mixtures prepared by Thrasyas of Mantinea, he stressed that, in Athens, hemlock only was used (without, thus, the addition of any other substance, toxic or not).

8.4 MODERN PHARMACOLOGICAL ANALYSIS

The silent and peaceful death of Socrates raises the question of whether hemlock has an analgesic effect. Until 2009, no information was available in the scientific literature. In 2009, Dayan [54] stated that "nociceptive responses were not affected" by poison hemlock. A pharmacological study conducted by Arihan et al. contradicted this statement [8], and proved 2000 years later that Galen's affirmation was pharmacologically sound. In this study, authors found that coniine, the active molecule of poison hemlock, shows analgesic activity at doses of 10 mg/kg and more prominently at 20 mg/kg in two well-established tests, namely the hotplate and writhing tests. Beyond this dose, lethality was observed. Additional information about potentiation was also presented in this publication, as morphine and coniine potentiate their analgesic activity when administered together [8].

8.5 TOWARD A RENEWED INTERPRETATION

On the basis of unanimous ancient documentation (be it related to Socrates' death or not, and be it technical or literary), *Conium maculatum* L. was known in antiquity. All sources provide clear evidence, though scant and fragmentary, of the use of *Conium maculatum* L. as an agent for the execution of humans condemned to death. The plant is considered to have a *cooling* property (just like sleep and death, which are characterized by a reduction of or the loss of the active principle of life). The symptoms of the internal absorption of *kôneion* are precisely described as a gradual loss of sensory perception with increasing asphyxia, gasping, loss of consciousness, and, finally, respiratory arrest.

The clinical signs in the report of Socrates' death in Plato's *Phaedo* indicate a paralysis proceeding from the feet to the abdomen and then through the chest. Death was caused by the cessation of respiration due to the paralysis of the diaphragm muscles.

It has to be noted that none of the signs considered to be typical of the absorption of opium in ancient medical and toxicological literature appears in the clinical description of the death of Socrates by Plato or in the works of the other individuals whom we have mentioned. This confirms the findings of the ancient texts, in which no mention of opium is made, as Lewin already noticed.

Some elements of the description of death by absorption of hemlock (be it the death of Socrates or of other individuals) require further consideration, principally the repeated mention in the texts above (particularly those of Seneca, Galen, and Aelian) of a cold gradually spreading through the body, and rigidity. These phenomena suggest a loss of peripheral sensation in the lower extremities [54], since Socrates could not feel the mechanical stimulus by the man who gave the poison. Cold should probably be interpreted on the basis of subsequent literature as a loss of painful stimulus, that is, analgesic activity.

However, some symptoms typical of the ingestion of hemlock (vomiting, dizziness, or loss of cognitive functions) do not appear, either in Plato's report [54] or in some of the other cases. The fact that Socrates covered his face with a sheet and no longer communicated with his pupils could explain why such typical symptoms were not mentioned: most of these symptoms (particularly dizziness and loss of cognitive functions) would not have been visible and thus would not have been noticed by Socrates' pupils, who were gathered around him. On the other hand, these symptoms (except vomiting) are clearly mentioned in Nicander's *Alexipharmaca* and in the treatise *On poison* ascribed to Dioscorides.

The study by Arihan et al. constitutes the first assessment of the analgesic activity of coniine on organisms. The analgesic activity of coniine was significant in doses close to lethal, and it may have been supplemented by a strong analgesic agent such as morphine in the case of the mixture prepared by Thrasyas of Mantinea and reported by Theophrastus.

The pharmacological assessment of the activity of coniine and opium suggests different analgesic mechanisms. Morphine is an agonist for central opiate receptors for analgesic activity, whereas coniine stimulates the nicotinic receptors [7,55]. Analgesic activity was possibly enhanced due to their different modes of action. Theoretically, coniine and opium combine well for a painless execution, as Thrasyas of Mantinea probably already understood in the fourth century BC.

8.6 CONCLUSION

According to our results, the report of Socrates' death made by Plato seems realistic. Since coniine exerts antinociception more strongly at doses close to lethal, Socrates probably felt no pain after he ingested the poisonous mixture made of hemlock. In addition, the statement by Theophrastus about hemlock and opium as ingredients of a toxic potion composed by Thrasyas of Mantinea may also be true, since these two agents complement each other in antinociception.

REFERENCES

[1] Boissier E. Flora Orientalis sive enumeratio plantarum in Oriente a Graecia et Aegypto ad Indiae fines hucusque observatarum. Geneva and Basel: H. Georg; 1872.

[2] von Stoerck A. Libellus, quo demonstratur: cicutam non solum usu interno tutissime exhiberi, sed et esse simul remedium valde utile in multis morbis, qui hucusque curatu impossibiles dicebantur. Vindobonae: J.J. Trattner (English translation: An essay on the medicinal nature of hemlock: in which its extraordinary virtue and efficacy, as well internally as externally used, in the cure of cancers... are demonstrated. London); 1760.

[3] Giseke AL. Ueber das wirksame Princip des Schierlings *Conium maculatum*. Arch Apotheker-Vereins 1827;20:97−111.

[4] Hoffmann W. Zur Kenntniss der Coniin-Gruppe. Ber Dtsch Chem Ges 1881;18 (5−23):109−31.

[5] Moore B, Row R. A comparison of the physiological actions and chemical constitution of piperidine, coniine and nicotine. J Physiol 1898;22:273−95.

[6] Forsyth CS, Speth RC, Wecker L, Galey FD, Frank AA. Comparison of nicotinic receptor binding and biotransformation of coniine in the rat and chick. Toxicol Lett 1996;89:175−83.

[7] Bowman WC, Sanghvi IS. Pharmacological actions of Hemlock (*Conium maculatum*) alkaloids. J Pharm Pharmacol 1963;15:1−25.

[8] Arihan O, Boz M, İskit AB, İlhan M. Antinociceptive activity of coniine in mice. J Ethnopharmacol 2009;125(2):274−8.

[9] Bowie E. Aelianus [2]. In: Cancik H, Schneider H, editors. Brill's New Pauly. Encyclopedia of the Ancient World, vol. 1. Leiden and Boston: Brill; 2002. p. 200−1.

[10] Schofield AF. Aelian, on the characteristics of animals, with an English translation, in three volumes. I Books I−V. Cambridge, MA/London: Harvard University Press/W. Heinemann; 1971.

[11] Furley WD. Andocides. In: Cancik H, Schneider H, editors. Brill's new pauly. Encyclopedia of the ancient world, vol. 1. Leiden and Boston: Brill; 2002. p. 677−8.

[12] Maidment KJ. Minor attic orators in two volumes. I antiphon, andocides, with an English translation. Cambridge, MA/London: Harvard University Press/W. Heinemann; 1982.

[13] Nesselrath H-G. Aristophanes [3]. In: Cancik H, Schneider H, editors. Brill's new pauly. Encyclopedia of the ancient world, vol. 1. Leiden and Boston: Brill; 2002. p. 1125−32.

[14] Rogers BJ. Aristophanes in three volumes. II The Peace, The Birds, The Frogs. With an English translation. Cambridge, MA/London: Harvard University Press/W. Heinemann; 1979.

[15] Jones WHS, Potter P, Withington ET. Hippocrates with an English translation. Cambridge, MA/London: Harvard University Press/W. Heinemann; 1923−2010.

[16] Potter P. Hippocrates [6] of Cos. In: Cancik H, Schneider H, editors. Brill's new pauly. Encyclopedia of the ancient world, vol. 6. Leiden and Boston: Brill; 2005. p. 354−63.

[17] Meister K. Diodorus [18] Siculus. In: Cancik H, Schneider H, editors. Brill's new pauly. Encyclopedia of the ancient world, vol. 4. Leiden and Boston: Brill; 2005. p. 444−5.

[18] Oldfather CH. Diodorus of Sicily, with an English translation, in twelve volumes, VI. Books XIV−XV.19. Cambridge, MA/London: Harvard University Press/W. Heinemann; 1963.

[19] Runia DT. Diogenes [17] Laertius. In: Cancik H, Schneider H, editors. Brill's new pauly. Encyclopedia of the ancient world, vol. 4. Leiden and Boston: Brill; 2004. p. 452−5.

[20] Hicks RD. Diogenes Laertius, lives of eminent philosophers with an English translation, in two volumes. Cambridge, MA/London: Harvard University Press/W. Heinemann; 1980.

[21] Touwaide A. Pedanius [1] Dioscorides. In: Cancik H, Schneider H, editors. Brill's new pauly. Encyclopedia of the ancient world, vol. 10. Leiden and Boston: Brill; 2007. p. 670−2.

[22] Wellmann M. Pedanii Dioscuridis Anazarbei, De materia medica libri quinque, 3 vols. Berlin: Weidmann; 1906−14.

[23] Beck LY. Pedanius Dioscorides of Anazarbus, De materia medica. Translated. Hildesheim/Zürich/New York, NY: Olms-Weidmann; 2005.

[24] Touwaide, A. Les deux traités toxicologiques attribués à Dioscoride. La tradition manuscrite du texte grec, édition critique et traduction, vol. 5. (PhD thesis), Louvain-la-Neuve: 1981.

[25] Touwaide A. L'authenticité et l'origine des deux traités de toxicologie attribués à Dioscoride. I. Historique de la question. II. Apport de l'histoire du texte. vol. 38. Janus; 1983. p. 1−53.

[26] Touwaide A. Les deux traités de toxicologie attribués à Dioscoride: Tradition manuscrite, établissement du texte et critique d'authenticité. In: Garzya A, editor. Tradizione e ecdotica dei testi medici tardo-antichi e bizantini. Atti del Convegno internazionale, Anacapri, 29−31 ottobre 1990. Naples: D'Auria; 1992. p. 291−339.

[27] Nutton V. Galen of pergamum. In: Cancik H, Schneider H, editors. Brill's new pauly. Encyclopedia of the ancient world, vol. 5. Leiden and Boston: Brill; 2004. p. 654−61.

[28] Kühn KG. Claudii Galeni opera omnia. Volumen XII. Leipzig: Knobloch; 1826.

[29] Kühn KG. Galeni opera omnia. Volumen VII. Leipzig: Knobloch; 1824.

[30] Grant M. Galen on food and diet, vol. 51. London: Routledge; 2000. p. 114.

[31] Fantuzzi M. Nicander [4] of Colophon. In: Cancik H, Schneider H, editors. Brill's New Pauly. Encyclopedia of the Ancient World, vol. 9. Leiden and Boston: Brill; 2006. p. 706−8.

[32] Gow AD, Schofield AF. Nicander, the poems and poetical fragments. Edited with an introduction, translation and notes. Cambridge: Cambridge University Press; 1953.

[33] Szlezák TA. Plato [1]. In: Cancik H, Schneider H, editors. Brill's New Pauly. Encyclopedia of the Ancient World, vol. 11. Leiden and Boston: Brill; 2007. p. 338−52.

[34] Fowler HN. Plato in twelve volumes. I. Euthyphro, Apology, Crito, Phaedo, Phaedrus, with an English translation. Cambridge, MA/London: Harvard University Press/W. Heinemann; 1914.

[35] Fowler HN. Plato in twelve volumes. III. Lysis, Symposium, Gorgias, with an English translation. Cambridge, MA/London: Harvard University Press/W. Heinemann; 1925.

[36] Sallmann K. Plinius [1]. In: Cancik H, Schneider H, editors. Brill's New Pauly. Encyclopedia of the Ancient World, vol. 11. Leiden and Boston: Brill; 2007. p. 383−90.

[37] Rackmann H, et al. Pliny, Natural history, with an English translation. Cambridge, MA/London: Harvard University Press; 1938−62.

[38] Baltes M. Plutarchus [2]. In: Cancik H, Schneider H, editors. Brill's New Pauly. Encyclopedia of the Ancient World, vol. 11. Leiden and Boston: Brill; 2007. p. 410−23.

[39] Perrin B. Plutarchus' Lives, with an English translation, in eleven volumes, VIII. Cambridge, MA/London: Harvard University Press/W. Heinemann; 1969.

[40] Dingel J. Seneca [2]. In: Cancik H, Schneider H, editors. Brill's new pauly. Encyclopedia of the ancient world, vol. 13. Leiden and Boston: Brill; 2008. p. 271−8.

[41] Basore JW. Seneca in ten volumes, I Moral Essays in three volumes. I. Cambridge, MA/London: Harvard University Press/W. Heinemann; 1970.

[42] Gummere RM. Seneca in ten volumes. VI Ad Lucilium Epistulae Morales with an English translation. Cambridge, MA/London: Harvard University Press/W. Heinemann; 1971.

[43] Harmon R. Theophrastus. In: Cancik H, Schneider H, editors. Brill's New Pauly. Encyclopedia of the Ancient World, vol. 14. Leiden and Boston: Brill; 2009. p. 508–17.

[44] Hort A. Theophrastus, Enquiry into plants and minor works on odours and weather signs with an English translation, in two volumes. Cambridge, MA/London: Harvard University Press/W. Heinemann; 1916–26.

[45] Schütrumpf EE. Xenophon. In: Cancik H, Schneider H, editors. Brill's New Pauly. Encyclopedia of the Ancient World, vol. 15. Leiden and Boston: Brill; 2010. p. 824–33.

[46] Brownson CL. Xenophon in seven volumes. I. Hellenica, Books I–IV, with an English translation. Cambridge, MA/London: Harvard University Press/W. Heinemann; 1968.

[47] Sibthorp J. Florae Graecae Prodromus: sive Plantarum omnium enumeratio quas in provinciis aut insulis Graeciae invenit. London: Typis Richardi Taylor, veneunt apud J. White; 1806–13.

[48] Amigues S. Théophraste, Recherches sur les plantes. Tome V: Livre IX. Paris: Belles Lettres; 2006.

[49] de Halacsy E. Conspectus florae Graecae, vol. 1. Leipzig: W. Engelmann; 1901.

[50] Boissier E. Supplementum florae Graecae. Leipzig: W. Engelmann; 1908.

[51] Flora Europaea. Rosaceae to Umbelliferae, vol. 2. Cambridge: University Press; 1968.

[52] Hegi G. Illustrierte Flora von Mittel Europa, V.2. Munich: J.F. Lehmanns; 1925.

[53] Lewin L. Die Gifte in der Weltgeschichte. Toxikologische, allgemeinverständliche Untersuchungen der historischen Quellen. Berlin: J. Springer; 1920.

[54] Dayan AD. What killed Socrates? Toxicological considerations and questions. Postgrad Med J 2009;85:34–7.

[55] Guyton A, Hall J. Textbook of medical physiology. Philadelphia, PA: W.B. Saunders Company; 2001. p. 556.

CHAPTER 9

The Oracle at Delphi: The Pythia and the *Pneuma*, Intoxicating Gas Finds, and Hypotheses

Jelle Zeilinga de Boer

Delphi's sanctuary lies cradled on the southern flank of Mount Parnassus and overlooks the Pleistos river valley. Archeological remains suggest that the oracular site dates back to the Mycenaean period when Gaia (Mother Earth) was worshipped. By the eighth century BCE the cult of Apollo (god of prophesy) had been established and Delphi developed into a Panhellenic cradle of religion that also regulated politics, relationships between city states, and public and private affairs. Its zenith, when pilgrims from across the Mediterranean world came for advice, lasted more than a thousand years, from ca. 700 BCE until 361 CE when Oribasius, sent to Delphi by Emperor Julian, reported that the well-built hall had fallen and the speaking waters were stilled. A few years later Eunapius wrote, "To all intelligent men the end of the temples... was painful indeed" [1].

Ancient literary texts with information about the oracle's workings include testimonies by a philosopher (Plato), historians (Diodorus and Pliny), poets (Aeschylus and Cicero), geographers (Pausanias and Strabo), and the famous essayist/biographer Plutarch, who served as high priest at Delphi. Strabo (64 BCE−25 CE) contributes:

> They say that the seat of the oracle is a cave that is hollowed out deep down in the earth, with a rather narrow mouth, from which rises a pneuma (gas, vapor or breath) that inspires a divine frenzy; and that over the cleft is placed a high tripod, mounting which the Pythian priestess receives the pneuma and then utters oracles in both verse and prose [2].

Plutarch (46−120 CE) left several accounts of the activities at the oracle and describes the relationship between Apollo and the Pythia as that of a musician and his instrument. He tells us that the *pneuma* was emitted "as from a spring" in the *adyton* (reserved and restricted inner sanctum) and scented like sweet perfume. Priests and consultants could on some occasions detect the aroma of the *pneuma* in the antechamber

History of Toxicology and Environmental Health. DOI: http://dx.doi.org/10.1016/B978-0-12-800045-8.00010-1

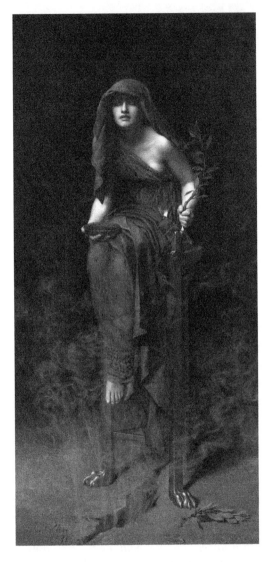

*John Collier, Britain, 1850–1934, (*Priestess of Delphi, *1891, London, oil on canvas, 160.0 × 80.0 cm, Gift of the Rt. Honourable, the Earl of Kintore 1893, Art Gallery of South Australia, Adelaide)*

where they waited for the Pythia's responses. Plutarch mentions that during his tenure, emissions had become weaker and more irregular. He suggests that either the vital essence had run out or that heavy rains in the mountains had diluted it. Earthquakes, he proposes, might have partially blocked the mouth of the cave, thus causing reduced flow. His hypotheses indicate a remarkable understanding of the hydrology and geology of the area! [3]

Pausanias (ca. 110–180 CE) writes about seeing a spring (the Kerna?) emerge on the slope above the temple and had heard that it plunged underground and emerged in the *adyton*, "where its waters made the priestesses prophetic" [4].

Oracular sessions were held on Apollo's Day, the seventh day after each full moon in spring, summer, and fall. The oracle did not operate in the winter months. Pilgrims would travel for weeks, mostly by boat, disembark at Kirrha, and climb the steep path to the oracle. Once there, they had to participate in several ritual procedures and wait their turn. If they missed sessions, or were passed over by more important patrons, they had to wait a full month or longer. During that time they could, and no doubt did, exchange information on the socioeconomic and political conditions in their kingdoms, cities, or towns. This was valuable material for the priests, who became well aware of the goings-on in their Mediterranean world. One wonders whether such intelligence may have colored their interpretations of the Pythia's responses during mantic services.

The Pythias were women from the village selected by the priesthood of the temple. Early in the morning on Apollo's Day, priests would lead the chosen priestess, who had been fasting for days, from her secluded home to the Kastalia spring. After purification, she would slowly and ceremoniously ascend the Sacred Way to the temple. Before entering she was offered a cup of holy water, obtained at the prophetic spring. After a few more ceremonies she would enter the temple and descend into its *cella* where the small *adyton* was located. After being seated on the tripod and given a few minutes to inhale the *pneuma*, the Pythia would go into a trance and the head priest would relay questions submitted by the visitors, who remained in a separate antechamber. During her trance, the Pythia spoke in altered voice and at times chanted her responses, on occasion indulging in wordplay, which the priests would decipher for the enquirer(s) to interpret.

Reconstructions of the *adyton* by Courby and Amandry suggest an asymmetric structure, vis-à-vis that of the temple that occupied a small space in the *cella* against its southeastern wall, below the site where the sixth column of the internal colonnade is believed to have been purposefully omitted during (re)construction in the fourth century BCE. The *adyton* was presumably covered by a low ceiling and measured about 2.90 m × 5.60 m. Inside stood a tripod and a beehive-shaped *omphalos* (the umbilicus of the earth) [5].

Since the volume of the *pneuma* that rose into the *adyton* presumably was small, there must have been a device that allowed for it to be concentrated. In September 1913, in the late stages of the long excavation process, a small *omphalos*-shaped relic appeared mysteriously inside the temple. French archeologists dismissed it as a modern base for a cross of the type commonly found on Christian shrines that had somehow slid inside the *cella*. Others, including Holland and the author, believe it to be genuine. This relic (28.7 cm high) is similar in shape and size to *omphaloi* depicted on bas-reliefs, coins, and ceramic wares from both the Classical and Hellenistic periods. It contains a square hole (3 cm × 4 cm wide) carved from top to bottom, widening downwards. Holland proposes that this funnel served to convey the inspiring fumes to the Pythia. In the month between successive mantic sessions, a simple cork would have allowed for as much as 300 mL of gas to accumulate inside this conduit and much more in the space carved out of its foot block [6].

The design of the Apollo temple is unique in all of Greece. First of all, it was constructed on a slope with abundant evidence for instability as the result of rock falls and landslides. Second, unlike most Greek temples, Apollo's realm had a recessed earthen *cella*. And third, a spring emerged inside as testified by the presence of thick travertine crusts and construction of a drainage tunnel leading through the southeastern retaining wall to the Fountain of the Muses. Clearly its design was based on a special need: the protection of a holy spring.

The orientation and setting of the temple has to do with the presence of a major, active fault, which is part of the many fractures that developed along the northern flank of the Corinth rift zone that cuts an east–west swath through central Greece. It is one of the most seismically active and rapidly extending areas in the world. Tectonic slip planes of the Delphi fault are exposed both east and west of the oracle site and their connection indicates that it passes at depth below the temple. With a tectonic recurrence periodicity of several centuries, segments of the crustal block south of this fault have slipped down a few meters at a time, causing earthquakes. Evidence of at least three historic ruptures can be recognized on the exposed fault planes. They might be related to destructive seismic events that occurred in the sixth century BCE (leading to construction of the Cyclopean wall), in 373 BCE, and in 83 BCE.

The Delphi fault intersects the Parnassus–Ghiona tectonic unit of the Hellinides, a massive complex of westward-thrusting limestone/dolomite slabs of the Cretaceous and Paleogene ages. The former were deposited in a shallow subtropical ocean and contain strata enriched in bituminous matter. In addition to this major east–west fault, swarms of older northwest- and northeast-trending fractures cut through the area. Groundwater rising along a concave segment of the Delphi fault emerges at the Kerna spring and continues downslope inside the northwest-trending Kerna fracture zone. Its presence inside the sanctuary is clearly shown by the linear arrangement of four extinct springs with travertine crusts.

In the late 1990s, an American team composed of a geologist (author), archeologist (Hale), and geochemist (Chanton) carried out an interdisciplinary study of the oracle site and Delphi region. The study included detailed analyses of the fault/fracture systems and the chemistry of the groundwater and travertine deposits. Sampling included travertine from inside the temple and thick crusts that had adhered onto the massive Ischegaon wall constructed after an earlier temple crumbled during the 373 BCE seismic events. These samples were found to contain small quantities of both methane and ethane. The highest concentrations were encountered in samples collected inside and near the southeastern wall of the temple. Commonly only very small volumes of gas are captured inside porous travertine deposits around active springs. The presence of hydrocarbon gases in the old crusts, however small, therefore indicates that significant volumes surfaced when this rock was formed [7].

Both ethane and methane were also encountered in water from the Kerna spring, as expected, in larger volumes. The Kerna water furthermore included trace amounts (7 nL/L) of ethylene. These discoveries led the researchers to conclude that hydrocarbon gases had emerged with groundwater in the *adyton* and that the gases likely represented the intoxicating vapors mentioned by the ancient sources [8].

The volume of water and gases that commonly surfaces along active faults varies significantly as a function of fault topography and recurring local as well as regional seismicity in the Gulf of Corinth rift zone. Brecciation during rupture and/or strong shaking opens fault zones and frequently increases their permeability. In March 1981, the author observed a major upwelling of gas in the Gulf of Alkyonides following rupture and seismic aftershock activity along a fault similar to the one at Delphi. Over time, newly opened spaces are slowly choked by the formation of calcareous crusts, which reduce or can even stop groundwater flow until seismic reactivation occurs. The present-day reduced flow of the Kerna spring is probably related to additional problems. Widespread deforestation and drainage of a large wetland on the southern flank of Mount Parnassus increased regional runoff and reduced groundwater penetration into bedrock.

In 2006, an Italian–Greek team of scientists (Etiope, Papatheodorou, Christodoulou, Geraga, and Favali) reappraised the natural gas occurrences at the oracle site. Their surveys included gas fluxes from soils, gas in groundwater, and isotopic analyses of the travertine deposits. They confirmed the earlier discovery of the hydrocarbon gases and concluded that methane, ethane, and carbon dioxide had been released from a thermogenic (catagenic) hydrocarbon source at depth, most likely bituminous enriched strata in the limestone complex. They found the highest methane flux in soils around the Kerna spring ($145 \, mg/m^2 \, d$). The soils in the temple *cella* contained $65 \, mg/m^2 \, d$. Kerna spring water yielded concentrations of $73.2 \, nmol/L$ methane and $2.2 \, nmol/L$ ethane. They found that the travertine crusts near the Kerna spring were formed mainly by oxidation of hydrocarbons to carbon dioxide, a process that also greatly facilitated the formation of thick travertine crusts elsewhere in the sanctuary.

The Italian–Greek team thus confirmed the surfacing of light hydrocarbon gases but did not believe that sufficient ethylene for inducing trancelike states in Pythias could have been produced in the deep carbonate rocks below Delphi, since that specific environment is not prone to biogenic production of ethylene. However, an abiogenic transformation of ethane to ethylene under thermal conditions generated by frictional heating in the fault zone during seismic rupture cannot be excluded. The team posited that the gas-linked neurotoxic effects could have resulted from oxygen depletion due to carbon dioxide/methane inhalation in the enclosed and nonventilated *adyton*. They also proposed that benzene, an aromatic hydrocarbon commonly dissolved in groundwater springs, might have been the culprit.

Short-term exposure to benzene, however, leads to shortness of breath, diminished mental alertness, and impaired vision. It also causes emotional instability. No such effects are reported to have commonly occurred in Delphi's long history [9].

During his long tenure at Delphi, Plutarch described only one instance in which a Pythia was not responding properly. He wrote, "She was like a laboring ship and was filled with a mighty and baleful spirit. Finally she became hysterical and with a frightful shriek rushed toward the exit" [10].

Scientists working at substance abuse centers have reported that all three gases—ethylene, ethane, and methane—can potentially produce an altered mental state. In present-day inhalant abuse, light hydrocarbon gases, due to their intoxicating properties, remain the primary sought-after substances. Ethylene, an aliphatic hydrocarbon gas with a sweet odor, is the most likely candidate for inducing a trance. A major advantage of ethylene is its lack of respiratory and cardiovascular depressing effects. Ethane would be nearly as potent. A mixture of the two would produce a significant altered state [11].

Ancient accounts have provided relatively clear descriptions of the Pythia in trance, namely that of a woman who willingly entered the *adyton*, remained conscious, and was able to respond to questions with visions described in tones and patterns of altered speech. Recovery was said to be rapid, and other than an out-of-body experience—the feeling of being possessed by the god Apollo—the Pythia would not remember events that had occurred while in trance. These effects are similar to those described by twentieth- and twenty-first-century toxicologists for patients under mild ethylene-induced anesthesia and thus add another level of congruency to reconcile contemporary science with classical wisdom concerning the Pythia and the *pneuma* [12].

When French archeologists began to excavate ancient Delphi in the 1890s, they first had to remove the modern settlement of Kastri, which had been built on top of the ruins. After exhaustive labor they unearthed the temple foundations but did not find a clear trace of the *adyton*. Furthermore, finding no evidence for a cave—and detecting no gases—they concluded that the ancient references must be erroneous. Unfortunately, their assumptions invaded principal textbooks, such as those by Parke and Fontenrose, and became dogmatic among scholars for much of the twentieth century [13].

In 2007, classicists Foster and Lehoux published a criticism of the Delphic ethylene intoxication hypothesis and concluded that the Pythias' behavior could not be accounted for by ethylene intoxication, because insufficient volumes rose into the *adyton*. No substantiation for this statement, other than referring to the hypothesis of Ethiope and colleagues, was provided. Continuing in its century-old vein, their criticism no longer centers on the possibility of vapors having risen in the inner sanctum, but on their volume: "Οσο πιο πολύ αλλάζουν τα πράγματα, τόσο παραμένουν ίδια!" (The more things change, the more they stay the same!) [14].

The ancient belief in intoxicating gaseous emissions at the site of the Delphi oracle is not a myth. An unusual, but by no means unique, combination of faults, bituminous limestone, and rising groundwater worked together to bring volatile hydrocarbon gases to the *adyton*. Contemporary geologic research has thus reaffirmed many if not most aspects of the ancient sources.

REFERENCES

[1] Philostratus (the Athenian), Eunapius. Philostratus and Eunapius: the lives of the Sophists, 427. London/New York, NY: William Heinemann, G. Putnam's Sons, MCMXXII.

[2] Strabo. Geography, 9.3. New York, NY: Putnam's Sons; 1927.

[3] Plutarch. De defectu oraculorum. Moralia, 437, 497–499. Cambridge, MA: Harvard University Press; 1936.

[4] Pausanias. Description of Greece, vol. 4. Cambridge, MA: Harvard University Press; 1935.

[5] Courby F. Fouilles de Delphes, tome II, Topographie et Architecture. Paris: E. de Boccard; 1927. Amandry P. La mantique Apollonienne A Delphes; Essai sur le functionnement de l'oracle. Paris: E. de Boccard; 1950. Amandry P. Recherches sur la cella du temple de Delphes. In: Heintz JG, editor. Oracles et propheties dans L'Antiquite: Actes du Colloque de Strasbourg 15–17 juin 1995, vol. 15. Paris: E. de Boccard; 1997. p. 215–30.

[6] Bousquet J. Observations sur l'omphalos archaique de Delphes. Bulletin de Correspondance Hellenique 1951;75:210–30. Holland LB. The mantic mechanism at Delphi. Am J Archaeol 1933;37:201–14. Zeilinga de Boer J. Delphi's small omphalos: an enigma. Syll Class 2007;18:81–104.

[7] Zeilinga de Boer J. Dilational fractures in the Corinthian and Evian rift zones. Annales Tectonicae 1992;6:41–61. Zeilinga de Boer J, Hale JR. The geological origins of the oracle in Delphi, Greece. In: McGuire B, Griffiths D, Steward I, editors. The archaeology of geological catastrophes, vol. 171. London: Geological Society of London, Special Publication; 2000. p. 399–412. Zeilinga de Boer J, Hale JR, Chanton J. New evidence for the geological origins of the ancient Delphic oracle (Greece). Geology 2001;29(8):707–10.

[8] Hale JR, Zeilinga de Boer J, Chanton JP, Spiller HA. Questioning the Delphic oracle. Sci Am 2003;8:67–73. See [7].

[9] Etiope G, Papatheodorou G, Christodoulou G, Geraga M, Favali P. The geological links of the ancient Delphic oracle (Greece): a reappraisal of natural gas occurrences and origin. Geology 2006;10:821−4.

[10] Plutarch. Plutarch; De defectu oraculorum, V: 499−500. Moralia. Cambridge, MA: Harvard University Press; 1936.

[11] Spiller HA, Hale JR, Zeilinga de Boer J. The Delphic oracle: a multidisciplinary defense of the gaseous vent theory. Clin Toxicol 2002;40(2):189−96. Dorsch RR, De Rocco AG. A generalized hydrate mechanism of gaseous anesthesia, 1. Theory. Physiol Chem Phys 1973;5:209−23.

[12] Spiller HA, Hale JR, Zeilinga de Boer J. The Delphic oracle: a multidisciplinary defense of the gaseous vent theory. Clin Toxicol 2002;40(2):189−96. Broad WJ. The oracle. The lost secrets and hidden message of ancient Delphi. New York, NY: The Penguin Press; 2006.

[13] Oppe AP. The chasm at Delphi. J Hell Stud 1904;24:214−40. Parke HW. A history of the Delphic oracle. Oxford, UK: Blackwell; 1939. Parke HW, Wormell DEW. The Delphic oracle. The oracular responses, vol. 2. Oxford, UK: Blackwell; 1956. p. 436. Fontenrose J. The Delphic oracle, its responses and operations. Berkeley, CA: University of California Press; 1978.

[14] Foster J, Lehoux D. The Delphic oracle and the ethylene-intoxication hypothesis. Clin Toxicol 2007;45(1):85−9. Lehoux D. Drugs and the Delphic oracle. Class World 2007;10(1):41−56. Etiope G, Papatheodorou G, Christodoulou G, Geraga M, Favali P. The geological links of the ancient Delphic oracle (Greece): a reappraisal of natural gas occurrences and origin. Geology 2006;10:821−4.

RECOMMENDED READING

Broad WJ. The oracle: the lost secrets and hidden message of ancient Delphi. New York, NY: The Penguin Press; 2006.

Lipsey R. Have you been to Delphi? Albany, NY: State University of New York Press; 2001.

CHAPTER 10

The Ancient Gates to Hell and Their Relevance to Geogenic CO_2

Hardy Pfanz, Galip Yüce, Francesco D'Andria, Walter D'Alessandro, Benny Pfanz, Yiannis Manetas and George Papatheodorou

10.1 INTRODUCTION

In Greek mythology, the world is divided into three realms. Zeus rules heaven, Poseidon the sea, and Pluto the shadows of the underworld. Since time immemorial, the living world was separated from the world of death, shadows, and souls. The underworld (hell, the netherworld, or Hades) was located either in remote astronomic regions or hidden somewhere in the underground. Those who had received proper burial rites were allowed to enter. This means that for those who have passed away, there must be a proper way to get there. In Greek mythology, the dead had to cross a certain river(s)—Acheron, Cocytus, Lethe, Styx, or Phlegeton.

Within the everlasting darkness there were many chthonian divinities, gods and goddesses considered the rulers of the underworld in classical mythology: the king of the netherworld was Pluto (note that there are various ways of spelling this name), Hades (Ἅδης, Haides, Aides, Ἀιδης), Aidoneus, Klymenos, Clymenus, Dis Pater, Orcus, and the goddesses Persephone, also known as Kore or Proserpina. Hades is the Lord of the Shadows, the King of the netherworld, the god of the lower world, and the sender of death to the mortals. Hades is also the god of funeral rites. He is mostly seen with his three-headed hellhound Kerberos (Latin: Cerberus). In the little book on images of the gods it is said that "...homo terribilis in solio sulphureo sedens, sceptrum regni in manu tenens dextra: sinistra, animam constringes, cui tricipitem Cerberum sub pedibus collocabant, et iuxta se tres Harpyias habebat. De throno aure eius sulphureo quatuor flumina manabunt, quae scilicet Lethum, Cocytu, Phlegethontem, et Acherontem appellabant, et Stygem paludem iuxta flumina assignabant."... This translates as "... an intimidating person sitting on a throne of sulfur, holding the scepter of his realm in his right hand, and with his left strangling a soul. Under his feet three-headed

History of Toxicology and Environmental Health. DOI: http://dx.doi.org/10.1016/B978-0-12-800045-8.00011-3

Cerberus held a position, and beside him he had three Harpies. From his golden throne of sulfur flowed four rivers, which were called, as is known, Lethe, Cocytus, Phlegethon, and Acheron, tributaries of the Stygian swamp" (as cited in Ref. [1], but see Refs. [2–5]).

There are two names for the entrances to hell: **Charonion** ([6], Strabo XIV, 1, 11) for the cave of Thymbria, between Magnesia on Maeander and Myus; and for Acharaka near Nysa on Maeander ([6], Strabo XIV, 1, 45–47) and **Ploutonion** for Hierapolis ([6], Strabo, XIII, 4, 14). *Plutonium* clearly means a sanctuary for the chthonic god Pluto, whereas Charonion refers to the ferryman Charon.

Extraordinary and fearsome places were often thought to be the entrance to the netherworld [7]. Caves, fissures, and fractures with smelly exhalations, and lakes or streams that were steaming hot or that changed color were such sites. The entrance to the underworld was sometimes also the end of the world. Odysseus was ferried there by Charon, across the River Styx, to find Tiresias ([8] Homer; Cantus XI; Odyssey). Quite a few ancient gates to hell are caves (see Ref. [7] and references therein) some others are lakes or depressions. Caves are uncertain places, entrances to a dark and unknown world. These places were even more fearful when, in addition to the darkness, toxic vapors were emitted, able to kill all life. The vapors were called mephitic vapors[1] which resembled the deadly Hadean breath (or the breath of the hellhound Kerberos). In most cases, these vapors consisted of highly concentrated carbon dioxide (CO_2), sometimes with some sulfur gas (H_2S) impurities. In geothermal fields or when hot water streams were present, large amounts of water vapor were emitted which led to the fearsome appearance of toxic mists and fogs in front of the cave.

The gate to the underworld was always thought to be related to supernatural forces and thought to be miraculous. In some cases, entrances to the Hadean underground may have been found by shepherds or herdsmen who witnessed their cattle behaving strangely at such places. Herdsmen were astute in observing nature; even a slight change or variation in the normal vegetation could alert them to such extraordinary places [9–11]. Corpses of small animals also hinted at the presence of strange and supernatural forces. If priests came to

---

[1]From Mefitis or Mephitis, a goddess of the evil geogenic smells, who was worshipped in Pompeii, Rocca San Felice or Rome.

know about such places, they declared them sacred. Sometimes temples and sanctuaries were built in the surroundings (or even on top of geogenic gas emissions; see Plutonium in Hierapolis/Phrygia).

Ustinova [12] mentioned that ancient Greek oracular cults focused on caves and suggested that the Greeks used at least two methods of divination. The easiest was sensory deprivation since the reduction of external stimuli leads to dream-like states. The second technique was based on special geological conditions, namely, a source of poisonous gas having euphoriant or psychotropic effects.

Dante Alighieri [13] was most probably the first to relate mythic places and geology (Cantus XII; XIV and XV). He describes the circum-volcanic conditions quite precisely and, not knowing the proper geologic interrelations, he ascribes them to hell. In modern times, B. Vitaliano was probably the first to use the term *geo-mythology* [14]. She was followed by Piccardi and Masse [15]. In the following remarks, we try an amalgamation of mythological and archeological data with geological, biological, and medical evidence to describe the coherence of the *geo-bio-mythology* of the ancient gates of hell.

10.2 WHY ENTER THE REALM OF THE SHADOWS?

10.2.1 The Souls of the Mortals

For humans who had passed away, the passage to the kingdom of the dead was probably not difficult, if their relatives took enough care during the funeral. The correct funeral procedure was an important aid and also a guarantee of sorts for a safe journey into the underworld. In Greek mythology, the souls of the dead, "the shadows," had to cross the river Styx (Acheron). The transfer across the Acheron via ferry was done by Charon, the ferryman of the shadows, who was paid by the "danakes (oboli)," mostly with golden coins that were put into the mouths of the dead before the funeral.

10.2.2 Incubation and Cure

The cult of worshipping Pluto was probably imitated from the cults of Serapis in Egypt [16]. Strabon (Book XIV) [6] mentions three sites in Asia Minor where Pluto was worshipped. In the region of Nysa and Acharaka he describes a temple for Pluto and Kore, as well as a grotto (the Charonion). Somewhere in the vicinity is Limon (λειμών, the meadow), where similar rites were practiced [16]. As a third

Plutonium, Strabo mentions the famous Hierapolis with its hot water ponds, its calcareous hot water falls (nowadays Pamukkale), and its Charonion (Strabon XIV). Pilgrims prayed for health and cure and/or asked for prophecies. Priests dealt with the gods of the underworld. The priests, rather than the patients, incubated, i.e. immersed themselves in the natural environmental phenomena of the site. The patients subsequently followed the recipes and cures that were prescribed according to the dreams of the priests during incubation. The prerequisites of prophecies and dreams were among other parameters (drugs, hallucinogenic plants, and mushrooms) attributed to the presence of geogenic gases. Lack of oxygen and an increase in carbon dioxide can cause hallucinogenic effects in humans (see also Ref. [17]). In this context, a theory has been proposed linking the prophetic power of the Pythia in Delphi's Sanctuary with the occurrence of gases released from a fault ("chasma") [17−19]. The Delphi Sanctuary is considered the most important religious location of the ancient Greek world ("omphalos" of the world). The sacredness of the oracle mostly centered on the mantic faculty of the Pythia, whose prophecies had a vital role in the political, social, and military scenes of the ancient world. De Boer et al. [17] proposed that the inhalation of the sweet-smelling ethylene, which can cause mild narcotic effects, could be the reason for the inspiration of Pythia. Etiope et al. [18] propose that if any gas-linked neurotoxic effect of the Pythia needs to be invoked, as suggested by historical tradition, it could be searched for in the possibility of oxygen depletion due to CO_2-CH_4 exhalation in the nonaerated inner sanctum ("adyton").

10.2.3 Necromancy

Only a few extremely brave heroes like Odysseus and Orpheus dared to make their way down to the netherworld. Orpheus did so to free his wife Eurydike, who had died from a snake bite and for Odysseus it was one of his twelve tasks. Necromancy is a technique to negotiate with the gods of the netherworld or to communicate with the shadows of the deceased. Odysseus wanted to enter the realm of the shadows to meet the ghost of the seer Teiresias. Kirke helped him by instructing Odysseus in the art of necromancy. According to Homer, these rites were performed on the borders of the underworld, near Tainaron (Cape Matapan). Other authors claim that Odysseus visited the Nekromanteion at the Acheron River (NW Greece) or even in Cumae (Campi Flegrei, southern Italy).

10.2.4 The Gate for Chthonic Gods and Ghosts of the Darkness

The gates to the netherworld were used not only by the dead and shadows or those seeking cures, but also by the gods of the netherworld themselves to step out onto the earthly upper world (and down again). The abduction of Persephone/Kore is very common in Graeco-Roman mythology. Hades came from the subterranean darkness to abduct and rape Persephone and to take her as his wife and as the Queen of the netherworld. Homer describes the descent to Hades with Kore as taking place in Nysa−Acharaka (Phrygia). Yet, some authors still think also Hierapolis may play a role. In a Roman version, known as the rape of Proserpina, Pluto abducts Proserpina at the Lago di Pergusa, located in the center of Sicily close to the town of Enna. In this case, the lake was selected not because of its magmatic gas emissions but because of its biogenic sulfur emissions and its color change to purplered. The red coloration of this circular pond was a hint regarding its chthonic forces [20,21].

10.3 THE GEOLOGIC BACKGROUND

10.3.1 Geogenic Gas Emission—Volcanoes, Faults, and Seismicity

In geodynamically active areas, which are characterized by intense volcanic activity and/or high seismicity and tectonics, many geogenic gases can be released to the atmosphere depending on the local geologic regime [22]. Among the major gas species, CO_2 is found in almost all of these areas. Water vapor is found in volcanic and geothermal areas where temperatures at or close to the surface reach the boiling temperature of water. Among sulfur gases, hydrogen sulfide (H_2S) is typical of geothermal areas while sulfur dioxide (SO_2) is released with high-temperature volcanic gases. The latter can also contain significant quantities of halogens, mainly in the form of HCl, HF, and HBr [23]. All remaining gas species, although relevant for geochemical studies (CO, noble gases, and hydrocarbon gases) and/or for their possible long-term effects on human health (Hg, Rn), are found only at trace levels. The only exception is geogenic CH_4, whose emissions may be relevant in sedimentary basins with petroleum production [24].

Concerning the gases measured around or within the gates to hell, CO_2 is, aside from water vapor, the most frequently found gas.

As mentioned above, geogenic gas emissions can lead to enhanced carbon dioxide concentrations that influence and threaten life in the area. Carbon dioxide of geologic origin is formed within the Earth's mantle or crust and is released to the atmosphere not only by volcanoes but also diffusely from the soil in geothermal areas. Gases reach the Earth's surface through zones of enhanced vertical permeability within the crust such as volcanic conduits, volcano-tectonic structures, and faults. In particular, faults generally act as important pathways for migration to the surface of carbon dioxide originating from deep thermo-metamorphism of carbonate rocks or mantle degassing [25,26]. When the gas leaves the lithosphere–pedosphere system, it reaches the adjacent atmosphere, where it is normally diluted due to convection triggered by sun or wind. Heavier than air, carbon dioxide can accumulate and reach high levels in valleys, depressions, and poorly ventilated zones and become dangerous for organisms. The reason is the specific density of CO_2 gas, which is 1.5 times heavier than air. This phenomenon is also known from wine cellars, where the fermentative CO_2 gas accumulates at the cellar bottom creating a potentially lethal trap for the wine makers. Some valleys or dolines (sinkholes) are well known for their dangerous gas atmosphere (Kies et al., unpublished, [10,27]). Such gas-filled depressions are known all over the world. In Rwanda they are called "mazuku" (evil wind). Carcasses of reptiles, birds, gorillas, and even elephants are sometimes found in their close vicinity [28]. Soentgen [11] also describes the possible relation between the gates to hell and places of oracles and geogenic gases.

10.3.2 Hot Water, Steam, and Geysers

Aside from toxic gas emissions there is also another geologic reason for the selection of sacred sites. Geothermal energy in hot water creeks, hot water steam, hot water eruptions (geysers), and the reddening of water bodies drew the attention of laypeople and ancient priests alike. Red water bodies can have an abiotic and a biotic cause. The red color of a creek is mainly due to the oxidation of reduced iron from great depths; iron oxides and hydroxides are formed (iron ochre). Such places were called "Bullicame" (bubbling water) in the Italian language of the Middle Ages. The term was used either for all stained hot water emanations or specifically for a little geothermal lake and creek close to Viterbo (Dante Alighieri, L'Inferno; Canto XII, 127–129) [13]. The physicochemical action of carbon dioxide to displace and withdraw oxygen is here precisely described. With Dante, CO_2 merely extinguishes flames; with Strabon it extinguishes human lives (see later).

10.4 THE PHYSICOCHEMICAL PROPERTIES OF CO_2

10.4.1 Carbon Dioxide is Difficult to Recognize

In contrast to heavily odorous gases like HCl, SO_2, or H_2S, carbon dioxide is described as colorless, odorless, and tasteless in its gaseous form [29].[2] This means that if an animal walks into a CO_2 gas cloud which is gradually increasing in concentration, it will not recognize the danger and become asphyxiated [30,31]. On the other hand, if one enters a region with a distinct and immediate transition of normal air to a concentrated CO_2 gas, the sudden change will clearly be noticed (see below).

10.4.2 Carbon Dioxide Forms Gas Lakes

The molecular weight of CO_2 is 44 g/mol. With its density of 1.98 kg/m^3, CO_2 is 1.5 times heavier than air [32]. Lower lying areas, holes, valleys, depressions, or even cellars will thus be filled with the gas and stable gas lakes can be formed [10,27,33]. Under calm weather conditions, such gas lakes form a very distinct boundary between the highly concentrated CO_2 gas lake and the above-lying atmospheric air. CO_2 concentrations can be as high as 80% within the gas lake and 0.5% in the direct vicinity of the boundary. Some centimeters distant, CO_2 concentrations drop to normal values of 0.04%. At the same time, oxygen concentrations may increase from 2% to 3% within the deadly gas lake to 20.9% in the adjacent atmosphere layered on top of the lake. According to what was said above, stable boundaries can easily be recognized by animals and can therefore be avoided. Gas lakes which would continuously increase in concentration would be a much larger threat to life. On the other hand, if organisms are trapped within such gas lakes they will lose consciousness within seconds to minutes and then die.

The density of CO_2 also leads to the formation of distinct gas creeks. In the geothermal area of the Sousaki volcano (Greece), two

---

[2]This is only partly true. If you try to inhale CO_2 concentrations of 35% and higher (don't do this because it is dangerous!), there is the sensation (smell and taste) of champange or mineral water. The champange-feeling is easily explained by the extremely high CO_2 concentrations that built up during opening of the bottle.

caves emit high amounts of CO_2 gas ($>90\%$ CO_2 within the cave) and a continuous gas creek flows out of the cave's mouth and downhill (Figure 10.1). On its way downhill it kills smaller organisms like mice, birds, and insects in its small riverbed.

It must be added that CO_2 gas lakes are stable only as long as no wind or sun action occurs. This is true for the Hadean grottos below the Apollo temple and the Plutonium in Hierapolis. It is also true for shady valley structures, CO_2 caves (aragonite cave at Zbrasov, Czechia), and for cellars and other basements of buildings. In all other cases, wind turbulence or convection created by solar irradiation will destroy the lake and form normal atmospheric conditions during sunny hours [10,27,33].

10.4.3 Carbon Dioxide Displaces Atmospheric Oxygen

Because of its presence in high concentrations, CO_2 displaces oxygen and in consequence aerobically breathing organisms will experience respiratory problems. As the highest possible oxidized state of carbon, CO_2 additionally is nonflammable and can thus be used to quench flames. This physical property of CO_2 is well known to firefighters, who extinguish fires by displacing oxygen using nonflammable CO_2. Dante Alighieri [13] described the extinguishing flames on the hot Bullicame creek (Canto XII, XIV, and XV).

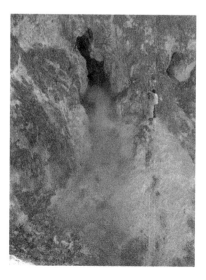

Figure 10.1 Dry CO_2 creek creeping out of a CO_2 cave at the crater rim of Sousaki volcano in Greece. The gas is heavier than air and flows downhill. The gas was stained with an orange smoke capsule.

10.4.4 Carbon Dioxide Forms an Acid

Gaseous CO_2 is the anhydride of carbonic acid. Furthermore, it is highly soluble in aqueous solutions. Once dissolved, carbonic acid dissociates according to Eq. (10.1), liberating one or two protons.

$$CO_2 + H_2O \leftrightarrow H_2CO_3 \leftrightarrow H^+ + HCO_3^- \leftrightarrow 2H^+ + CO_3^{2-} \qquad (10.1)$$

Liberation of protons leads to an acidification of the aqueous phase. Depending on the actual buffering capacity, acidification may be larger or smaller [34,35]. Aqueous phases exist on surfaces and also within organisms. The liquid film on eyes, the mucosae in the nose and lung, and all intercellular compartments are prone to the acidifying effect of CO_2. Itching of these body parts or the inhibition of enzymatic action may be the consequence [36].

10.5 THE BIOLOGICAL, MEDICAL, AND PHYSIOLOGICAL BACKGROUND

High concentrations of CO_2 can act in two ways: (i) on the one side, high carbon dioxide concentrations displace atmospheric oxygen, and (ii) on the other side, CO_2 is potentially acidic and deprotonates in solution. In the first case, the physiological effects are hypercapnia, or oxygen deficiencies like hypoxia or even anoxia. In the latter case, cellular compartments become acidified [36] and enzyme action is reduced or blocked [35].

Therefore, extreme CO_2 concentrations cannot be tolerated by aerobically breathing creatures (Figure 10.2); anaerobic organisms (e.g., some bacteria and archaea), on the other hand, would survive. So clearly, oxygen-dependent life—mammals, reptiles, and birds—could not have existed within the grotto of the Plutonium in Hierapolis (Pfanz et al. unpublished). Even insects would have been killed within minutes (for some exceptions see Ref. [37]). Mammals already react to CO_2 concentrations as low as 3−5% [30,31,38]. Even these rather low concentrations may increase cardiac and respiratory rates if exposure time is longer than several minutes [10,39−41]. At CO_2 concentrations around 8−10% humans are asphyxiated; longer exposure at 15−20% inevitably leads to death. A detailed list of human reactions to different CO_2 concentrations is found in the IVHHN Gas Guidelines [42].

Divers have to cope with oxygen deficiencies and an overdose of CO_2 in their blood. Pregnant women can use a trick during the birth

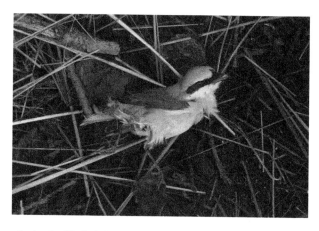

*Figure 10.2 An asphyxiated red-backed shrike (*Lanius collurio*) in a small depression in a mofette meadow in Czech Republic.*

process to manipulate their blood pH: re-inhaling expired CO_2 (folding the hands in front of the mouth) leads to a decrease in blood pH whereas panting alkalizes the blood. In this way, strong pain can be reduced and the oxygen level necessary for mother and baby is conserved. Sudden infant death syndrome (SIDS) is sometimes related to hypercapnia.

Too much CO_2 leads to dizziness. There are reports of miners digging for coal and lignite who were overcome by sudden leaks of CO_2. Similar fatalities are described for brewers and firemen [43].

The catastrophic events at Nyos and Monoun helped increase knowledge of CO_2 extremes [44]. In 1986, more than 1700 people died in a volcanic CO_2 gas accident. The Nyos volcanic crater lake was supersaturated with CO_2 that leaked from its base into the water [45]. Cold temperature and a high water pressure (due to a water depth of 253 m) led to a supersaturation of the lake water with carbon dioxide. Due to an earthquake with a concomitant landslide the surplus of gas was spontaneously set free and a 30-m-high gas cloud was formed upon the lake surface. Due to its special density this deadly gas cloud flowed downhill through a narrow valley, reaching several villages and killing 1700 people and 5000 cattle. Many of the corpses looked like they were sleeping. Only few had blisters and a bigger skin rash. The latter were thought to be due to *rigor mortis* and concomitant changes, because the victims were found several days after the accident [46]. Similar CO_2 accidents due to volcanic CO_2 exhalations have been reported from Lake Kivu, Nyiragongo, Djeng Plateau, and many other places [28,40,47].

The positive CO_2 effects are fewer but nevertheless worth mentioning. The correct concentration of CO_2 in breathable air may enhance blood circulation. Patients with low blood pressure and concomitant cold limbs therefore take "dry CO_2 baths" to speed up circulation [48]. At CO_2 concentrations between 25 and 35% (w/v), the hands and feet of elderly people warm up within a few minutes. Care has to be taken, however, that the deadly gas atmosphere is not directly inhaled. Patients simply stand in a 1- to 1.2 m-high, dry CO_2 gas lake. In several countries (Romania, Bulgaria, Hungary, and Slovakia) dry CO_2 gas cures are well known and some health resorts are famous for their geogenic gas (e.g., Harghita Mountain in Romania; [49]).

Not only blood circulation is affected. There are also verbal records of the positive effects of high CO_2 levels on skin diseases caused by bacteria and fungi. The potentially acidic action of CO_2 in aqueous phases [35] and within cells may reduce the viability of the pathogens, leading to relief of pain. The effects of warm mineral- and CO_2-containing cure waters are well documented.

Whether these positive effects of geogenic CO_2 gas were actually used in front of the Plutonia has not yet been studied in detail. Yet, the rites of incubation and the rituals around prophecies and seeing strongly hint in this direction [17,50].

10.6 ACTUAL GAS CONCENTRATIONS AROUND AND WITHIN GATES TO HELL

The existence of deadly vapors (*spiritus letalis, mantikon pneuma*, and *anathymiasis*) around the gates of hell is described by several authors. "Foramina pestilens exhalatur vapor ..." can be read in Seneca [51] (Naturales Quaestiones, libro VL, Chapter 28). But Plinius [52] (Historia naturalis), Strabon [6], and Virgilius [53] (Cantus VI, Aeneis) also mention a deadly haze around Plutonia and Charonia (see also Refs. [7,11]). The extremely high CO_2 concentrations and the concomitant low oxygen concentrations within the Hadean antechambers (grottos) below the theatron in the Plutonion and the Apollo temple in Hierapolis/Phrygia are highly toxic. Outside the subterranean grotto, in front of the stone benches, solar irradiation and wind do not allow a persistent gas lake. Yet, the permanent flow of CO$_2$ out of the chamber onto the floor of the theatron forms a transient gas lake. As with many other CO$_2$ gas lakes, the toxic atmosphere forms in the evening hours, persists throughout the night, and is reduced in the morning due to the absorption by the infrared portion of sunlight [10,33,50]. The great number of corpses of insects and birds prove its existence: dead birds and more than 70 dead beetles (Tenebrionidae, Carabaeidae, and Scarabaeidae) were found asphyxiated on the floor. Locals report on dead mice, cats, weasels, and even asphyxiated foxes. Most of them weren't killed during sunny days, but during the dark hours. Insects are the exception: they were seen to be asphyxiated even during midday hours. Even then, a thin 5 cm "high CO$_2$ gas layer" covered the ground in front of the grotto of the Plutonium at Hierapolis, killing smaller beasts.

In Mefite D'Ansanto, Chiodini et al. [54] measured a total output of about 1000 t of CO$_2$ per day over an area of 4000 m^2. Such a huge CO$_2$ output is not connected to volcanic activity but the C and He isotopic composition of the gases points to the same mantle origin of the nearby volcanic systems of Vesuvius and the Phlegrean Fields. The massive output together with the right topographic situation allows the build-up of sometimes lethal conditions at the main venting area and along the narrow valley immediately downstream. Chiodini et al. [54] found that in the absence of wind, the lethal concentration of 15% of CO$_2$ at 1.5 m height extends for about 200 m along the valley, while the dangerous threshold of 5% at the same height extends for more than 1 km, reaching far beyond the area devoid of vegetation. It is therefore not hard to believe that at least 12 persons died from the gas at this site between the seventeenth century and the present [54].

10.7 THE KNOWN SITES OF ANCIENT GATES TO HELL

In principle, the existence of ancient gates to hell reflects the ancient realm of Greece and its colonies (Magna Graecia and Asia Minor). The entrances to the netherworld are known for southern Italy, for the Greek mainland, and for the Asia Minor part of modern Turkey.

10.7.1 Italy (Magna Graecia)

Within the modern borders of Italy, gates to hell may be found in the larger region around Mount Vesuvius. Here many craters of the

Phlegrean Fields (with mofettes, solfatares, and fumaroles), the volcanic lakes of Averno and Agnano, and also the Grotta del Cane and Mefite D'Ansanto can be found. For the Grotta del Cane and other gas caves in the vicinity the so-called *spiritus letalis* (deadly haze) is mentioned [11].

10.7.1.1 The Phlegrean Fields (Campi Flegrei)
Bordering the gulf of Naples and in sight of Mount Vesuvius, the caldera of a super-volcano is located. The region of the Campi Flegrei (burning fields) is punctuated by several volcanoes, older calderas, volcano lakes, and gas-emitting vents [55]. The whole area is additionally prone to bradyseismism, meaning that the whole region has an uplift of several meters and then slowly collapses. Within this area are the towns of Pozzuoli and Cumae and a large part of Naples.

10.7.1.1.1 Lago Averno
In the southern part of the Campi Flegrei close to the coast is the saline lake called Lago Averno. Its water composition is the result of the mixing of seawater and saline hydrothermal fluids [56]. At present, the input of gases is very low and the overturn of its waters depends only on temperature-driven density stratifications. Such overturns happen only in correspondence with particularly cold winters; many fish are killed due to the H_2S-rich and O_2-poor composition of the deepest layers. The H_2S is not only of hydrothermal origin but derives also from sulfate reduction in the deep anoxic part of the lake. The mass of the upwelled gas and the extent of the consequent fish-killing depends mainly on the length of the previous accumulation period [56].

In Roman times, this kind of overturn mechanism was less probable because the lake was opened to the sea and transformed into the main military port hosting the imperial fleet. In such conditions, it was less probable that the surface layers would become denser, triggering an overturn of its waters. It cannot be excluded that at that time hydrothermal gas inflow or CH_4 production in the deeper anoxic parts was higher, leading to bubbles rising or even lake overturn.

Several ancient writers expect the Lago Averno to be a gate to hell. Gas emissions are also mentioned: "No bird is able to fly over its surface but will soon die because of toxic vapors" [53]. The name Averno is derived from *aornos*, meaning "birdless" in Greek. In the vicinity, the Roman hero Aeneas met Sybilla to ask her for the way to meet his father (Virgil, Aeneis, Cantus VI). She explains that it is easy to find the way to Pluto right through the Lake Averno. Several times Virgil mentions toxic exhalations from the lake that killed all life.

10.7.1.1.2 Solfatara and Pisciarelli

More or less in the center of the Phlegrean Fields directly belonging to the settlement of Pozzuoli, the large crater of Solfatara resembles a hostile, nonhabitable place on earth. Many mofettes and solfatares emit toxic gases in addition to fumarolic hot water emissions [55]. Due to the wide and open morphology of the area, CO_2 does not generally reach dangerous levels but concentrations of a few hundred parts per million in excess of normal atmospheric air at 1.5 m height even at daytime testify to the strong CO_2 emission [57]. The contemporaneous release of other typical hydrothermal gases (water vapor and hydrogen sulfide) contributes to the image of an entrance to hell. According to Capacio [58] and Galanti and Jagemann [59], the caldera of Pozzuoli was thought to be the market square in front of the hell and the abysm to hell (Figure 10.3).

10.7.1.2 Bullicame

Dante Alighieri [13] described the extinguishing flames on the hot creek Bullicame close to Viterbo (L'Inferno, Canti XII, 127–129, XIV, 88–90 and XV, 1–3). He describes this geothermal phenomenon, with additional degassing of sulfurous and carbonic gases, in his song of the

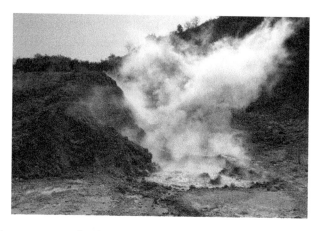

Figure 10.3 Hot water steam and carbon dioxide emanating from a bubbling pool at Pisciarelli (close to Solfatara) in the Phlegreian Fields, Pozzuoli, Italy.

hell as "…a hot stream of blood and sulfur.…" Although not directly knowing the type of gas, Dante clearly describes the physical action of highly concentrated carbon dioxide clouds:

Cosa non fu dagli occhi tuoi scorta
Notabil come lo presente rio,
Che sopra sè tutte fiammelle ammorta.

Nothing has been discovered by thine eyes
So notable as is the present river
Which all the little flames above it quenches.

(L'Inferno, Canto XIV, 88–90)

10.7.1.3 Mefite D'Ansanto
In Virgil (Book VII) [53] it is written:

[565]*est locus Italiae medio sub montibus altis,*
nobilis et fama multis memoratus in oris,
Amsancti valles; densis hunc frondibus atrum
urget utrimque latus nemoris, medioque fragosus
dat sonitum saxis et torto vertice torrens.
hic specus horrendum et saevi spiracula Ditis
monstrantur, ruptoque ingens Acheronte vorago
pestiferas aperit fauces, quis condita Erinys,
invisum numen, terras caelumque levabat.

(Virgil Aeneis, Book VII)

Approximately 80 km east of Mount Vesuvius there is a place now called *Mefite D'Ansanto*, the epitome of all CO_2 degassing sites. In the area the goddess Mefitis (Mephitis) was worshipped. For Virgil this place is the entrance to the underworld (Aeneis, Book VII). CO_2 degassing is so strong here that the pond at the base bubbles heavily and within 20,000 m^2 no vegetation can be found (Figure 10.4). Naked soil, void of any life, covers the ground around the venting area. The degassing area is surrounded and framed by reed grass (*Phragmites australis*) and several *Juncus* and *Agrostis* species able to tolerate even peak concentrations of CO_2. The gas flow is so high that a dry CO_2 gas creek runs downhill, using the riverbed of an ephemeral creek. The area downhill is extremely dangerous to spectators of the mephitic sanctuary as wind gusts may blow deadly CO_2 gas parcels unexpectedly in any direction (see also Ref. [54]).

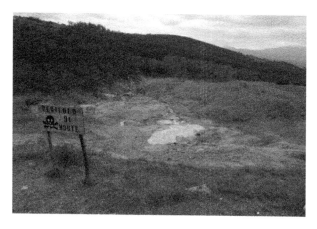

Figure 10.4 The eponymous CO_2 degassing mofette Mefite D'Ansanto in Southern Italy. The area is void of vegetation, indicating extreme CO_2 soil fluxes and concentrations.

10.7.1.4 Naftia

About 50 km southwest of Mt. Etna in Sicily is another strong CO_2 degassing site called Naftia, which has been compared by many authors to the Mefite D'Ansanto. This site has been known since ancient times; it was described by geographers like Strabo and Diodorus Siculus and more recently by Ferrara [60]. At this site abundant gas, mainly composed of CO_2, bubbled within a shallow lake. In the past, the lake generally dried out during summer, leaving two craters from which gas was continuously emitted. The lake has now been reclaimed and transformed into arable land; while gas emission still occurs [61], it has been strongly reduced by industries that use the gas.

This site must be considered a gate to the netherworld, since it is related to the chthonian deities of the Palikoi. Their mythological history can be found in the scripts of many ancient writers (e.g., Aeskylus, Virgil, Ovid) although in different versions.

The origin of the myth surely predates the Greek colonization of the inner part of Sicily. The Palikoi were previously adored by the indigenous Sikel population. Recent archeological investigations show that the site had been inhabited since the Neolithic age and that the building of a sanctuary started in the seventh to sixth century BC [62,63]. The Palikoi were the personification of the natural gas emission phenomenon. They were twins representing the two main gas emission points in the lake, which created two geyser-like columns; their "comeback" from the netherworld was certainly connected to the annual disappearance of the lake, which dried out in the summer, leaving two deep craters, and to their return in the rainy autumn−winter period typical of the Mediterranean climate.

The cult of the Palikoi lasted at least until the Roman imperial period and their sanctuary had great importance: it was the site of an oracle, an asylum for runaway slaves, and a place where oaths could be tested by different rituals. These rituals were tightly connected to the CO_2 degassing activity of the lake. In one version of the rituals, the oaths were written on tablets and thrown into one of the bubbling craters. If the tablet floated on the water, the oath was considered to be true, but if it sank, the oath was regarded as perjury. The destiny of the tablet strongly depended on the part of the water surface that it reached. In those parts where no gas came up or where the gas pressure was very high, the tablet was sustained above the water; where degassing activity was less, the bubbles would lower the water density and consequently the tablet would sink.

In another ritual, the person to be tested had to go close to the gas emission, and after making his oath, had to bow down and touch the crater. Depending on the degassing activity and on the meteorological conditions, he could be overwhelmed by the CO_2 and suffocate. This would have been interpreted as a sign of his perjury. In this case the punishment was seen as coming directly from the gods while in the previous case the perjurer was sentenced to blinding or death.

10.7.1.5 Lago di Pergusa

Not directly related to geogenic gas but probably due to biogenic sulfur gases is the gate to the netherworld at the Lago di Pergusa. Located in the center of Sicily near the town of Enna, this circular brackish lake regularly blooms with algae and bacteria. Semi-saline algae from the family Chromatiaceae (*Thiocapsa roseopersicina* and *Thiodictyon elegans*) are the cause of the red coloration [20]. According to Ovid [64] (Metamorphosis 5.385−391), it was later thought that the lake was one of the sites where Hades abducted Kore (Persephone/Prosperina). Close to the lake there are remnants of a temple devoted to Demeter/Ceres.

10.7.2 Greece

10.7.2.1 Eleusis—The Elysian Grotto

Probably the most important center where Demeter and her daughter Persephone (Ceres and Kore) were worshipped was the Plutonium of Eleusis in Attica (Elefsina in modern Greece). According to several authors this site is not only the gate to hell but the most important place where Pluto was thought to abduct and rape Persephone [65]. The Plutonium proper consists of two half-caves and a forecourt (Figure 10.5). On the right side of the half-cave there is a smaller cave and a hole through which Persephone annually escapes from Pluto's realm to reenter the desiccated earth at the end of Mediterranean summer. The appearance of Persephone makes her mother Demeter happy and therefore spring, with its concomitant sprouting and blooming, occurs.

Yet, although this Eleusian site is the well-documented *locus typicus* of a Hadean gateway, no degassing of CO_2 could be found within the cave and its surroundings (Pfanz and Manetas, 2013, unpublished).

10.7.2.2 The Nekromanteion of Acheron-Ephyra

The death oracle (Nekromanteion) of Acheron is located in the ancient region of Thesprotia (now Prevesa). The region was formerly a swampy area with several rivers and the lake Acherusia. Like Cape Tainaron (see below), it is thought that Kirke led Odysseus to the Hadean

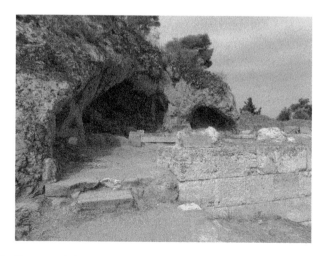

Figure 10.5 The Plutonium of Eleusis in Attica where Pluto was thought to abduct and rape Persephone. The proper Plutonium consists of two half-caves and a forecourt.

underworld to meet the seer Teiresias ([8] Homer, Odyssey; [66] Herodot 5, 92; [67]). Theseus was also thought to visit the underworld in Acheron. Close to the confluence of the Acheron (Periphlegeton) and Kokytos Rivers is a cave thought to be the abyss to Hades [67]. The waters of the rivers derive from the underworld river Styx. It is said that at a certain ford of the Acheron River, poplars and willows would grow but their fruits would die off (gas?). The ruins of the Nekromanteion are located west of the ancient lake Acherusia, close to the village of Mesopotamos. A small statue of Persephone was found and evidently proved that this was the proper site [67]. Yet, several authors deny that the ruins are related to the famous Nekromanteion; rather, they believe it to be an eighteenth-century monastic church [68].

10.7.2.3 Cape Tainaron

At the tip of the Mani peninsula in southern Peloponnes, there seems to be an alternative entrance to hell with which the shadows can avoid crossing the rivers Acheron or Styx. The death oracle is described as an entrance to hell by Ovid (Book X, Metamorphosis). Orpheus visited the underworld (Tartarus) via this gate. It was also at this entrance that Heracles, in his Twelfth Labor, confronted and captured the fierce three-headed hound, Kerberos, guardian of the gate. Geogenic degassing has not yet been studied at this place.

10.7.3 Turkey—Asia Minor

10.7.3.1 Hierapolis

In contrast to Eleusis, extreme CO_2 concentrations were found within and around the sanctuary of Hierapolis/Phrygia (Pamukkale, Turkey). Hierapolis is located in the Denizli Graben, which is a geological disturbance zone extending between the Pamukkale and Babadag faults. First recordings of the town were made by Strabo (XII, 8, 17), and Plinius the Elder (Nat. Hist. V, 105) also mentions it. The town, probably a Seleucid foundation in the third century, developed during the Roman Empire and was famous in Byzantine times. Hierapolis is cut longitudinally by several parallel fractures of the Pamukkale fault by intra-plate tectonics and was destroyed by many earthquake events [69−71]. Built directly upon this fault are two buildings: the famous Apollo temple [72] and the newly discovered Plutonium, the sanctuary of the Gods of the underworld, Hades and Kore, with the theater above a grotto [73]. Several sources mention that strange things happened at the outlet of the Plutonium. Priests demonstrated their supernatural power and their equality to the gods by ushering animals like goats and bulls into the antechamber where, after a short time, the animals showed signs of suffocation, finally dying after several minutes (Strabo XIII, 4, 14, Plinius, Nat. Hist. II, 207–208, and Ref. [7]).

10.7.3.1.1 The Plutonium

After the excavation conducted by D'Andria in 2011–2013, a subterranean grotto was found below the stone seats of the Theatron (Figure 10.6). The grotto belongs to the Sanctuary of Pluto and Kore. The words "Ploutoni kai Kore" in Greek letters engraved into the stone row are still readable. In front of the small hole of the grotto, dead insects and birds can be found.

Gas measurements inside the closed subterranean chamber (grotto) revealed CO_2 concentrations of up to 91%. The entire basement of the grotto was totally dark but seemed to be highly humid, due to a warm, carbonate-rich creek flowing below it. Deadly CO_2 gas also exists in front of the actual grotto. Flooding out of the grotto's mouth, the escaping CO_2 forms a gas lake on the floor. The corpses of animals hint at the absence of oxygen and the presence of high CO_2 that builds up during the night.

10.7.3.1.2 The Temple of Apollo

Similar findings were obtained when the grotto under the Temple of Apollo was studied. The sanctuary of Apollo is situated 200 m north

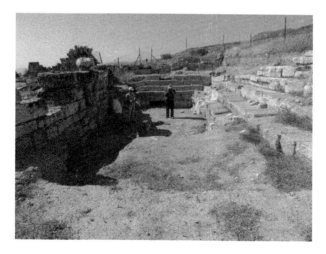

Figure 10.6 The Plutonium of Hierapolis in Phrygia during its excavation. The proper entrance to hell is on the right side, not yet excavated. Deadly high CO_2 concentrations (90%) were measured within the grotto below the seat rows.

of the Plutonium within the same seismic fracture zone and has long been known for its subterranean pit structure. This pit was interpreted as Plutonium in previous excavations and it is marked as such in touristic guides for Hierapolis. Recent excavation (2011−2013) has demonstrated that the Plutonium proper is located in the area south of the Apollo Sanctuary. The toxicity of its gas atmosphere is known and it has been therefore firmly walled for safety reasons. Within the mouth-hole of the Apollo−Plutonium, CO_2 levels between 60% and 65% were measured; at the same time oxygen was only 8−8.5%.

10.7.3.2 Nysa and Acharaka

Close to Acharaka and Nysa ad Maeandrum, there was another sanctuary of Pluto and Persephone and an additional Charonion. This site was well known for incubations and health cures. The abduction of Persephone is also thought to have occurred here. It has not yet been proven that CO_2 gases occur around the sanctuaries but sulfur-containing gases have been shown to escape from caves and from some creeks. Strabon (Geographica 14.144) also describes the sacrifice of bulls and other sacred animals. The detailed descriptions of the death of these animals are consistent with those reported for the Plutonium at Hierapolis.

10.8 THE HISTORICAL RELEVANCE

Several gates to hell are described in ancient literature, although few have been seriously checked for the occurrence of geogenic gas emissions. In some places, it has been clearly demonstrated that deadly high CO_2 emissions occur exactly as described by the ancient writers (Pfanz et al., unpublished). A *mantikon pneuma*, a prophetic mist or smoke from the soil, or an *anathymiasis* (an exhalation) is described by Plutarch, who was an eyewitness of the functionality of Delphi [11]. In Hierapolis/Phrygia, the source of this deadly gas is clearly the subterranean grotto, which is considered to be the entrance to the Hadean underworld (Plutonium, Charonion; Strabo XIII, 4, 14, Plinius, Nat. Hist. II, 207−208, and 7, 73). All these authors and many others describe the deaths of small birds that were sold by locals and bought by spectators and ancient visitors of the sanctuary. The animals were thrown into the gaseous atmosphere just below the seats of the theatron; spectators watched how they died [7]. Strabo and Plinius also describe the sacrifice of bulls or goats within the grotto. Priests demonstrated their supernatural powers and their equality to the gods by ushering animals like goats and bulls into the Plutonium. The authors describe exactly how the bulls showed signs of suffocation, how their bodies trembled, and how the otherwise robust herbivores died within minutes. Yet the Galloi, the castrated priests of the Mother Goddess (Cybele), survived (Strabo XIII, 4, 14, Plinius, Nat. Hist. II, 207–208, and [7]). These priests often stood on slightly elevated places. They knew about the deadly vapors. They probably also knew the exact height of the deadly gas lake. During the sacrifice of animals they tried not to breathe deeply [7].

The toxic atmosphere in front of the gates to hell was thought to resemble the deadly smell of hell's unpleasant atmosphere, but it was also attributed to the breath of the ferocious hellhound Kerberos. He was posted to prevent ghosts of the dead from leaving the netherworld. Several sources exist which describe the deadly smell from the mouth of this terrible, three-headed hell guard ([74] Pausanias, Description of Greece 2. 35.10). Even the saliva of this wild beast was poisonous. When Odysseus drove Kerberos out of Hades (which was one of his twelve tasks), the dog spat slime on the ground. From this toxic saliva the deadly toxic plant aconite, or wolf's bane (*Aconitum napellus*), was born (Hesiod, Theogony, 769 ff. and Ref. [75]). There is even a relation between the breath and slime of Kerberos and the hallucinogenic effects described in the neighborhood of the caves to hell: "... (the Erinys) Tisiphone brought with her poisons too of magic power (to invoke madness): lip-froth of Cerberus, the Echidna's venom, wild deliriums, blindness of the brain, and crime and tears, and maddened lust for murder; all ground up, mixed with fresh blood, boiled in a pan of bronze, and stirred with a green hemlock stick." (Ovid, Metamorphoses, 4.500 ff. and Ref. [75])

It seems that in ancient times natural phenomena mostly could not easily and satisfactorily be explained [76]. If they were additionally associated with pain and death, they were attributed to the deadly necrotic and chthonic forces living at unpleasant places of no return. The invisible haze resembled ghosts or gods or the breath of the ferocious hellhound. It was something unexplainable, something supernatural, and something fearsome. It can therefore be assumed that the ancient word for gas is god or death or mephitis. Nowadays these phenomena can easily be described and analyzed by physicochemical means and quantitatively explained with knowledge from geology, chemistry, and biology. It is surprising, however, how precisely and without exaggeration ancient writers were able to describe these exciting natural (or possibly supernatural) phenomena.

ACKNOWLEDGMENT

We want to thank the Governorship of Denizli city, the Director of Hierapolis/Pamukkale, and the provincial culture and tourism directorate of Ankara and Denizli. We would like to acknowledge the kind help of Dr. Kalliope Papaggeli (Director of Elefsina archeological site), Dr. Pio Panarelli, Dr. Kadir Özel, Dr. Marco Esposito (Hierapolis excavation site), Dr. Giovanni Chiodini, Dr. Stefano Caliro (Osservatorio Vesuviano, Napoli), and Dr. Antonio Raschi (CNR, Firenze).

REFERENCES

[1] Pluto Mythology: <http://www.en.wikipedia.org/wiki/Pluto_(mythology)>.

[2] Albricus Philosophus. De deorum imaginibus libellus. Chapter VI: De Plutone; 1742.

[3] Raschke R. De Alberico mythologo. Dissertation, University of Breslau; 1912.

[4] Wolf FA. In: Gürthler JD, Hoffmann SFW, editors. Vorlesungen über die Alterthumswissenschaft, vol. 3. Leipzig: Lehndholdsche Buchhandlung; 1839.

[5] Pepin RE. The Vatikan mythographers. Rome: Fordham University Press, 2008.

[6] Strabo XIV, 1, 11; XIV, 1, 45–47; XIII, 4, 14.

[7] Zwingmann N. Antiker Tourismus in Kleinasien und auf den vorgelagerten Inseln. Bonn: Habelt Verlag; 2012.

[8] Homer [c. 700 BCE]. The Odyssey [S. Butler, Trans.]. London, UK: Longmans, Green & Co; 1900.

[9] Pfanz H, Vodnik D, Wittmann C, Aschan G, Raschi A. Plants and geothermal CO_2 exhalations: survival in and adaptation to a high CO_2 environment. In: Esser K, Lüttge U, Kadereit JW, Beyschlag W, editors. Progress in botany, 65. Berlin/Heidelberg: Springer Verlag; 2004. p. 499–538.

[10] Pfanz H. Mofetten—kalter Atem schlafender Vulkane. Köln: RVDL-Verlag; 2008.

[11] Soentgen J. On the history and prehistory of CO_2. Found Chem 2010;12:137–48.

[12] Ustinova Y. Cave experiences and ancient Greek oracles. Time Mind 2009;2:265–86.

[13] Dante Alighieri. Die göttliche Komödie. Hölle. Leipzig: Faber&Faber; 2001.

[14] Vitaliano DB. Legends of the earth: their geologic origins. Bloomington, Indiana, USA: Indiana University Press; 1973.

[15] Piccardi L, Masse WB, editors. Myth and geology. London: The Geological Society; 2007.

[16] Hamilton M. Incubation—or the cure of disease in Pagan temples and Christian churches. St. Andrews: WC Henderson & Son; 1906.

[17] De Boer JZ, Hale JR, Chanton J. New evidence for the geological origins of the ancient Delphi oracle (Greece). Geology 2001;29:707–10.

[18] Etiope G, Papatheodorou G, Christodoulou D, Geraga M, Favali P. The geological links of the ancient Delphic Oracle (Greece): a reappraisal of natural gas occurrence and origin. Geology 2006;34:821–4.

[19] Piccardi L, Monti C, Vaselli O, Tassi F, Gaki-Papanastassiou K, Papanastassiou D. Scent of a myth: tectonics, geochemistry, and geomythology at Delphi (Greece). J Geol Soc 2008;165:5–18.

[20] Kondratieva EN, Zhukov VG, Ivanovsky RN, Petushkova YP, Monosov EZ. The capacity of phototrophic sulfur bacterium *Thiocapsa roseopersicina* for chemosynthesis. Arch Microbiol 1976;108:287–92.

[21] Rigoglioso M. Persephone's sacred lake and the ancient female mystery religion in the womb of Sicily. J Fem Stud Religion 2005;21:5–29.

[22] Hansell A, Oppenheimer C. Health hazards from volcanic gases: a systematic literature review. Arch Environ Health 2004;59:628–39.

[23] Aiuppa A, Baker DR, Webster JD. Halogens in volcanic systems. Chem Geol 2009;263:1–18.

[24] Etiope G, Klusman RW. Microseepage in drylands: flux and implications in the global atmospheric source/sink budget of methane. Global Planet Change 2010;72:265–74.

[25] Chiodini G, Frondini F, Kerrick DM, Rogie J, Parello F, Peruzzi LF, et al. Quantification of deep CO_2 fluxes from Central Italy. Examples of carbon balance for regional aquifers and of soil diffuse degassing. Chem Geol 1999;159:205–22.

[26] Mörner NA, Etiope G. Carbon degassing from the lithosphere. Global Planet Change 2002;33:185–203.

[27] Raschi A, Miglietta F, Tognetti R, van Gardingen PR. Plant responses to elevated CO_2. Evidence from natural CO_2 springs. Cambridge: Cambridge University Press; 1997.

[28] Vaselli O, Capaccioni B, Tedesco D, Tassi F, Yalire MM, Kasarerka MC. The evil winds (mazukus) at Nyiragongo volcano (Democratic Republic of Congo). Acta Vulcanol 2002/2003;14/15:123–8.

[29] Sax NI, Lewis RJ. Dangerous properties of industrial materials. 7th ed. New York, NY: Van Nostrand Reinhold; 1989.

[30] Krohn TC, Hansen AK, Dragsted N. The impact of low levels of carbon dioxide on rats. Lab Anim 2003;37:94–9.

[31] Niel L, Stewart SA, Weary DM. Effect of flow rate on aversion to gradual-fill carbon dioxide exposure to rats. Appl Anim Behav Sci 2007;109:77–84.

[32] Lide DR. CRC handbook of chemistry and physics. 84th ed. Boca Raton, FL: CRC Press; 2003.

[33] Bettarini B, Grifoni D, Miglietta F, Raschi A. Local greenhouse effect in a CO_2 spring in Central Italy. Ecosystems response to CO_2. The Maple Project results. Luxembourg: European Commission; 1999. p. 13–23

[34] Pfanz H, Heber U. Buffer capacities of leaves, leaf cells, and leaf cell organelles in relation to fluxes of potentially acidic gases. Plant Physiol 1986;81:597–602.

[35] Pfanz H. Apoplastic and symplastic proton concentrations and their significance for metabolism. In: Schulze E-D, Caldwell MM, editors. Ecophysiology of photosynthesis. Ecol Stud 100. Berlin/Heidelberg: Springer Verlag; 1994. p. 103–22.

[36] Pfanz H, Heber U. Determination of extra- and intracellular pH values in relation to the action of acidic gases on cells. In: Linskens HF, Jackson JF, editors. Modern methods of plant analysis NS. vol. 9. Gases in plant and microbial cells. Berlin/Heidelberg: Springer Verlag; 1989. p. 322–43.

[37] Russell D, Schulz H-J, Hohberg K, Pfanz H. The collembolan fauna of mofette fields (natural carbon-dioxide springs). Soil Org 2011;83:489−505.

[38] Hill L, Flack M. The effect of excess carbon dioxide and of want of oxygen upon the respiration and the circulation. J Physiol 1908;37:77−111.

[39] Ikeda N, Takahashi H, Umetsu K, Suzuki T. The course of respiration and circulation in death by carbon dioxide poisoning. Forensic Sci Int 1989;41:93−9.

[40] D'Alessandro W. Gas hazard: an often neglected natural risk in volcanic areas. In: Martin-Duque JF, Brebbia CA, Emmanouloudis DE, Mander U, editors. Geo-environment & landscape evolution II. Southampton: WIT Press; 2006. p. 369−78.

[41] D'Alessandro W, Kyriakopoulos K. Preliminary gas hazard evaluation in Greece. Nat Hazard 2013;69:1987−2004.

[42] IVHHN, International Volcanic Health Hazard Network. <www.ivhhn.org/gas/guidelines.html>.

[43] Baxter PJ. Hunter's diseases of occupations. In: Baxter PJ, Adams PH, Aw TC, Cockcroft A, Harrington JM, editors. Gases. London: Arnold; 2000. p. 123−78.

[44] Sigurdsson H, Devine JD, Tchoua FM, Presser TS, Pringle MKW, Evans WC. Origin of the lethal gas burst from Lake Monoun, Cameroun. J Volcanol Geotherm Res 1987;31:1−16.

[45] Rice A. Rollover in volcanic crater lakes: a possible cause for Lake Nyos type disasters. J Volcanol Geotherm Res 2000;97:233−9.

[46] Baxter PJ, Kapila M. Acute health impact of the gas release at Lake Nyos, Cameroon, 1986. J Volcanol Geotherm Res 1989;39:265−75.

[47] Le Guern F, Tazieff H, Faivre-Pierett R. An example of health hazard: people killed by gas during a phreatic eruption: Dieng Plateau (Java, Indonesia), February 20th 1979. Bull Volcanol 1982;45:153−6.

[48] Hadnagy C, Benedek G. Information of action mechanism of mofettes in Covasna. Arch Phys Ther 1968;20:229−33.

[49] Neda T, Szakacs A, Cosma C, Mocsy I. Radon concentration measurements in mofettes from Harghita and Covasna Counties, Romania. J Environ Radioact 2008;99:1819−24.

[50] Etiope G, Guerra M, Raschi A. Carbon dioxide and radon geohazards over a gas-bearing fault in the Siena Graben (Central Italy). TAO 2005;16:885−96.

[51] Seneca. Naturales Quaestiones, libro VL, Chapter 28.

[52] Plinius. Historia Naturalis, V, 105 and II, 207−208, and VII, 73.

[53] Virgilius Mar P. In: Fink G, editor. Aeneis. Düsseldorf: Artemis and Winkler; 2005.

[54] Chiodini G, Granieri D, Avino R, Caliro S, Costa A, Minopoli C, et al. Non-volcanic CO_2 earth degassing: case of Mefite D'Ansanto (southern Apennines), Italy. Geophys Res Lett 2010;37:L11303.

[55] Granieri D, Avino R, Chiodini G. Carbon dioxide diffuse emission from the soil: ten years of observations at Vesuvio and Campi Flegrei (Pozzuoli), and linkages with volcanic activity. Bull Volcanol 2010;72:103−18.

[56] Caliro S, Chiodini G, Izzo G, Minopoli C, Signorini A, Avino R, et al. Geochemical and biochemical evidence of lake overturn and fish kill at Lake Averno, Italy. J Volcanol Geotherm Res 2008;178:305−16.

[57] Carapezza M, Gurrieri S, Nuccio PM, Valenza M. CO_2 and H_2S concentrations in the atmosphere at Solfatara di Pozzuoli. Bull Volcanol 1984;47:287−93.

[58] Capacio JC. Puteolana historia. Napoli: C Vitalis; 1604.

[59] Galanti GM, Jagemann CJ. Neue historische und geographische Beschreibung beider Sicilien, vol. 4. Leipzig: Sigfried Lebrecht Crucius; 1793.

[60] Ferrara F. Memorie sopra il Lago Naftia nella Sicilia meridionale: sopra l'ambra siciliana sopra il mele ibleo e la città d'Ibla Megara sopra Nasso e Callipoli. Palermo: Dalla reale stamperia; 1805. p. 216

[61] De Gregorio S, Diliberto IS, Giammanco S, Gurrieri S, Valenza M. Tectonic control over large-scale diffuse degassing in eastern Sicily (Italy). Geofluids 2002;2:273–84.

[62] Maniscalco L, McConnell BE. The Sanctuary of the Divine Palikoi (Rocchicella di Mineo, Sicily): fieldwork from 1995–2001. Am J Archaeol 2003;107:145–80.

[63] Maniscalco L, editor. Il santuario dei Palici: un centro di culto nella Valle del Margi. Collana d'Area. Quaderno n. 11. Palermo: Regione Siciliana; 2008.

[64] Publius Ovidius Naso. Metamorphosis 5.385–391.

[65] Von Uxkull W. Die eleusinischen Mysterien. Versuch einer Rekonstruktion. Büdingen-Gettenbach: Avalun Verlag; 1957.

[66] Herodot 5, 92.

[67] Dakaris SI. Das Nekromanteion am Acheron. Athens: Zaravinos; 2001.

[68] Wiseman J. Rethinking the "Halls of Hades". Archaeology 1998;51:12–7.

[69] Hancock PL, Altunel E. Faulted archaeological relics at Hierapolis (Pamukkale), Turkey. J Geodyn 1997;24:21–36.

[70] D'Andria F, Silvestrelli F. Ricerche archeologiche turche nella valle del Lykos, Galatina; 2000.

[71] D'Andria F. Hierapolis of Phrygia (Pamukkale). An Archaelogical Guide, Pamukkale; 2003.

[72] Negri S, Leucci G. Geophysical investigation of the temple of Apollo (Hierapolis, Turkey). J Archaeol Sci 2006;33:1505–13.

[73] D'Andria F. Il Ploutonion a Hierapolis di Frigia. Istanbuler Mitteilungen 2013;63:157–217.

[74] Pausanias, Description of Greece—Greek Geography C 2nd A.D.

[75] Greek gods. <http://www.theoi.com/Khthonios/Haides.html>.

[76] Masse WB, Barber EW, Piccardi L, Barber PT. Exploring the nature of myth and its role in science. In: Piccardi L, Masse WB, editors. Myth and geology, 273. London: Geological Society; 2007. p. 9–28 [Special Publication]

CHAPTER 11

Lead Poisoning and the Downfall of Rome: Reality or Myth?

Louise Cilliers and Francois Retief

Lead, one of the seven metals of antiquity, has been mined since the fourth millennium BC. In the Graeco–Roman era, the use of lead increased remarkably and the metal probably became a health hazard to the population between 500 BC and 300 AD [1]. Pliny the Elder recognized the toxicity of lead, but the clinical picture of chronic lead poisoning was not clearly described. Despite this, there have been hypotheses that lead toxicity contributed significantly to the decline and fall of the Roman Empire [2].

In this study, the nature and extent of lead poisoning in ancient Rome is reviewed with emphasis on its possible influence on the long-term development of the region.

11.1 THE LEAD INDUSTRY IN ANCIENT ROME

11.1.1 Lead Production

Lead was originally mined from ores like *cerusite* (lead carbonate) and *galenite* (lead sulfide), which also contained silver, copper, gold, and even arsenic. Lead was produced in foundries near mines, and it is very probable that workers were exposed to extensive contamination from lead powder and fumes [3].

During the Roman era, lead production increased significantly. At its peak, the Roman Empire probably produced 80,000 tons of lead annually, comparable to two-thirds of the lead production in the United States in the 1970s. This amounts to approximately 4 kg of lead per capita annually [4].

Besides *cerusite* and *galena*, the Romans were aware of other lead products: *litharge* (lead oxide, yellow lead) was used in the building trade; *cerusa* (lead carbonate, white lead) was an industrial product,

History of Toxicology and Environmental Health. DOI: http://dx.doi.org/10.1016/B978-0-12-800045-8.00012-5

occasionally used as medicine; sugar of lead (lead acetate) was commonly used as sweetener, and in the preservation of wine and food [5].

11.1.2 Uses of Lead

The word "plumbing" is derived from the Latin *plumbum* (lead). In water conduits, lead was extensively used to line or seal earthenware pipes, aqueducts, tanks, and reservoirs. Domestic containers and cooking utensils commonly contained lead. Bronze and copper pots were frequently lined with lead (or a lead–silver alloy) to counter the unpleasant copper taste in the food. Lead provided a sweetish flavor. Pewter (lead and tin alloy) utensils were in common use. Containers for wine and olive oil were frequently made of lead or had a lead lining. Wine was commonly fermented in vats with a lead lining [6].

Sugar was unknown and honey was expensive. The Romans, thus, made common use of grape must concentrate as a sweetener. This was prepared by way of a cooking process, preferably in lead-lined copper pots, resulting in *sapa* or *defrutum*. This lead-contaminated product was used as a sweetener in food and wine, as a preservative in canned fruit, and as an inhibitor of fermentation in the wine industry. Lead acetate (sugar lead), prepared by adding acetic acid to lead, was also used as a sweetener.

Lead preparations (*cerusa*, lead carbonate, in particular) were used as facial powders, ointments, eye medicine, and white paint. It is also suggested that lead preparations were used for contraception, and the Roman botanist Dioscorides prescribed *litharge* for skin ailments; the medical use of lead has, however, remained limited through the ages. The Roman population also came in contact with lead in various other ways, for example, handling of lead ornaments; lead in roofing materials and gutters; coins; projectiles used in times of war; and in the shipping and building industry in general [7].

11.2 HUMAN EFFECTS OF LEAD

11.2.1 Metabolic Effect

Lead has extensive toxic effects on human tissue. It blocks enzymatic action (sulfhydryl radicals in particular) and has a direct toxic effect on organs such as the liver and kidney, as well as the nervous system, bone, hair, and hemopoietic organs. Lead is absorbed slowly through the skin but rapidly through the lungs and intestinal tract. In the body, redistribution of lead occurs and, eventually, 90% of that not excreted by the kidney accumulates in bones. Skeletal lead gives an indication of total lead absorption, and is not systemically toxic [8].

11.3 CLINICAL PICTURE OF LEAD TOXICITY [9]

Acute poisoning presents as abdominal pain, nausea and vomiting, painful mouth and throat with a metallic taste, thirst, and eventually diarrhea. Large doses may cause shock, peripheral paresthesia, pain, and muscular weakness. In severe cases, hemolytic anemia and renal failure may lead to death after a day or two.

Chronic poisoning presents with various symptom complexes: an abdominal syndrome with anorexia, a metal taste, gray "lead line" on the gums, severe constipation, and acute colic; a neuromuscular syndrome characterized by peripheral paralysis—for example, "wrist drop," asthenia, and encephalopathy (especially in children); a hematological syndrome with anemia due to bone marrow depression, or hemolytic anemia due to production of weak red blood cells. Gout may occur ("saturnine gout") due to renal damage. A characteristic pallor, unassociated with anemia, is also recognized.

11.4 ARCHAEOLOGICAL DETERMINATION OF LEAD TOXICITY

In children, lead toxicity manifests as diagnostic "lead bone lines" in x-rays, but this investigation is rarely used by archeologists [10].

Lead content of bone can be determined by atomic absorption spectrophotometric analysis, and gives an indication of the individual's total lead exposure during life. Possible contamination from soil surrounding the skeleton must be excluded. It is important to remember that bone lead will not increase during acute poisoning, and lead distribution is not uniform through the skeleton—it is higher in the skull, ribs, and vertebrae than in the pelvis and arm bones. For a comparable lead intake, bone lead is higher in children than adults, and in older specimens of bones compared to younger ones. Lead content of hair also reflects systemic lead load but is of limited value because of the brief lifespan of hair [11].

11.5 OCCURRENCE OF LEAD TOXICITY

11.5.1 Sources of Toxicity

We have convincing evidence that lead production and utilization increased significantly during Graeco–Roman times. According to some scholars, lead production in Europe and the Mediterranean area rose 10 times during the second millennium BC, to reach a peak by 500 BC. Subsequently, it decreased progressively up to 1000 AD, to reach levels similar to those of the third millennium BC [12].

Sources of lead contamination in Roman times may be summarized as follows:

- Domestic use of water from lead and lead-lined water conduits. It has, however, been postulated that this was a limited source of contamination, because flowing domestic water absorbs little lead from pipes; calcium precipitates from hard water would also have decreased contamination. The Roman architect, Vitruvius, however, claimed that water from earthenware pipes was healthier than that from leaden pipes. He also noted lead contamination of water originating from areas with mines and foundries.
- Lead from medicines and cosmetics would have caused toxicity only if consumed orally by intent or accidentally. Lead absorption through the skin is minimal [13].
- Contamination of food, wine, and olive oil due to preparation in pewter or lead containers, and addition of sugar lead (*sapa*) were important causes of lead poisoning. It has been calculated that 50–60% of a free adult Roman's lead intake probably came from wine. The nobility and the rich, who drank up to 2 L wine per day, would thus have been predisposed to lead poisoning. Pewter ware was extensively used by the middle class. It is calculated that the Roman aristocrat probably took in 250 mg of lead per day, the plebeian 35 mg, and the slave 15 mg. This compares with 30–50 mg of lead per day for the average contemporary adult in the United States. WHO considers 45 mg per day as the maximal lead intake for a healthy individual [14].

Workers in lead mines, foundries, and lead production works were prominently exposed to lead contamination. Approximately 80,000 laborers were annually exposed to contamination at lead works, and a further 60,000 at production units. Hygiene was primitive, although protective clothing for the head and face was in use, and probably protected against toxic inhalations. Pliny the Elder described the toxic effects of foundry gases on humans and animals [15].

11.5.2 Proof of Lead Poisoning
11.5.2.1 Clinical Picture
Ancient writers knew that lead products were poisonous. Dioscorides writes that *cerusa* taken orally was potentially fatal, and that certain sweet wines affected the abdomen and nerves negatively. Pliny the Elder commented on the poisonous nature of lead fumes, the toxicity of certain lead preparations, and the negative effect of *sapa*-containing wines on certain persons; the encyclopedist Celsus refers to the toxicity of white lead; Vitruvius wrote that lead pipes caused illness (but went on to design water conduits with prominent lead components) [16].

Nicander, a Greek poet of the second century BC, is generally credited for the first description of acute lead poisoning. This episode refers to an illness caused by *cerusa* (lead carbonate): acute abdominal upset, vomiting, painful muscles with progressive paralysis, involuntary eye movements, disturbed balance, hallucinations, and death.

However, chronic lead poisoning as we understand it was not clearly described in this era. Gout, which may be associated with chronic lead poisoning, was, of course, well described. The full classical description of chronic lead poisoning was by Paul of Aegina in the seventh century AD [17].

11.5.2.2 Archeological Findings [18]
Analysis of bone lead values relevant to the present study were reported by P. Grandjean. Additional analyses include those of Sudanese skeletons from as early as 3300 BC; prehistoric Danish skeletons; British skeletons from the Roman era; skeletons from the North American colonial era; Peruvian skeletons from 500–1000 AD; and European skeletons from the eighteenth century BC to the twentieth century AD.

Findings may be summarized as follows:

- With Sudanese and Peruvian data taken as "zero values" (from before the era of lead contamination), modern bone lead values represent a 20- to 100-fold increase.

- In spite of a wide intragroup variation, affluent communities showed higher lead concentrations than the poor, and urban communities higher concentrations than rural communities.
- During the late Roman period, lead concentrations in Roman occupied areas were 41–47% of contemporary levels in Europe. After 500 AD these values fell to 13% of modern levels, but during the Middle Ages they rose again to values comparable to the levels of ancient Rome.
- Lead levels in the capital, Rome, were not significantly higher than in legionary cities like Augsburg.

11.6 DISCUSSION

It is clear that the production and utilization of lead increased significantly from the second millennium BC to approximately 500 AD. This resulted in significant environmental lead contamination, and the question arises as to what extent this negatively affected the population of ancient Rome.

During the past century it has been suggested that lead contamination possibly hastened the decline and fall of the Roman Empire. It was speculated that lead poisoning specifically affected the aristocracy, diminishing their fertility and reproduction, and so decreasing Roman leadership. J.D. Nriagu and others argued that use of lead-contaminated water supplies, cooking procedures, and wine production specifically exposed the leaders to lead contamination.

Scarborough and Needleman and Needleman, however, warn that the extent of lead contamination should not be overestimated. While *sapa* prepared in lead containers undoubtedly contained much lead, lead containers were not necessarily used by the majority of the population. The amount of *sapa* added to wine was also not standardized. Pliny the Elder claimed that there were 185 types of wine in his day, each with its own composition. He preferred unsweetened wine. If sweetened wines were the most serious cause of lead poisoning, the extent of poisoning would thus depend on the distribution and use of types of wine [19].

Gilfillan believes that lead poisoning decreased fertility and caused miscarriages and abortion, thus precipitating the decrease in aristocracy evident from the first century BC. Aristocratic names like Julius and Cornelius, for instance, disappeared systematically. However, lead's actual influence on pregnancy is quite uncertain—only exposure to high doses of lead has been shown to affect pregnancy. Needleman and Needleman argue strongly that the actual cause of the gradual diminution of aristocratic family names and the decrease in family sizes is complex in nature, involving many factors besides possible lead contamination [20].

If lead contamination did in fact comprise a serious community problem in ancient Rome, the question arises as to why the typical clinical picture of chronic lead poisoning was not described, while the toxicity of lead was indeed appreciated. Nicander's poem describing acute lead poisoning appeared in the second century BC but Paul of Aegina's description of recognizable chronic poisoning did not appear until the seventh century AD. Vague descriptions of abdominal pain and muscular weakness by Pliny the Elder and Vitruvius do not constitute convincing evidence of the community's appreciation of lead poisoning. It is possible that gout, common in Roman times, could, however, have been a manifestation of subclinical lead poisoning.

Archeological evidence based on skeletal bone lead confirms that the mean lead content of the Roman population was less than half that of the modern European [21]. This does of course not mean that episodes of lead poisoning did not occur or that lead poisoning could not have occurred endemically in parts of the Empire. The affluent Roman took in more lead than the less privileged. Studies from Augsburg and Britain showed skeletal lead contents comparable with that of Rome. While lead contamination in antiquity was predominantly the result of oral intake, it was probably supplemented by pulmonary contamination from lead fumes in foundries. The high skeletal lead content of the modern European is the result of inhalation of lead-containing petrol fumes [9].

In summary, we accept that increased lead production occurred during the second millennium BC, reaching a peak during the Roman Empire. This caused significant contamination of the population and the affluent citizenry in particular. Although clinical lead poisoning probably occurred sporadically, archeological evidence indicates that the mean skeletal lead content of the population was less than half that of the modern European in the same countries. The typical clinical picture of chronic lead poisoning was not described before the seventh century AD.

It is thus unlikely that lead poisoning played a significant role in the decline and fall of the Roman Empire toward the fifth century AD.

REFERENCES

[1] Waldron T, Wells C. Exposure to lead in the ancient populations. Trans Stud Coll Physicians Phila 1975;1:102–15. Drasch GA. Lead burden in prehistorical, historical and modern human bodies. Sci Total Environ 1982;24:199–231.

[2] Retief FP, Cilliers L. Loodvergiftiging in antieke Rome (Lead poisoning in ancient Rome). Acta Acad 2000;32(2):167–84.

[3] Nriagu JO. Occupational exposure to lead in ancient times. Sci Total Environ 1983;32:105–16. Gilfillan SC. Lead poisoning and the fall of Rome. 1965;7:53–60.

[4] Woolley DE. A perspective of lead poisoning in antiquity and the present. Neurotoxicology 1984;5(3):353–61. Needleman L, Needleman D. Lead poisoning and the decline of the Roman aristocracy. Classical Views 1985;29:64–94.

[5] Waldron & Wells [note 1] p. 102–15. Waldron HA. Lead poisoning in the ancient world. Med Hist 1973;17:391–9; Pliny. Natural history [Rackham H, Trans.]. Loeb Classical Library. Cambridge MA: Harvard University Press; 1956. vol. 7, c.50.

[6] Needleman & Needleman [note 4] p. 64–94; Waldron [note 5] pp. 391–9.

[7] Gilfillan [note 3] p. 53–60; Pedanius Dioscorides of Anazarbus. De materia medica [Beck LY, Trans.]. Olms: Weidman; 2005, Bk. V.87.

[8] Drasch [note 1] p. 199–231; Retief & Cilliers [note 2] pp. 167–84.

[9] Retief & Cilliers [note 2] pp. 167–84.

[10] Jarcho S. Lead in the bones of pre-historic lead-glaze potters. Am Antiq 1964;30(1):94–6. Waldron & Wells [note 1] pp. 102–15.

[11] Grandjean P. Widening perspectives of lead toxicity. Environ Res 1978;17:303–21. Drasch [note 1] pp. 199–231.

[12] Nriagu [note 3] pp. 105–16.

[13] Nriagu [note 3] pp. 105–16; Retief & Cilliers [note 2] pp. 167–84; Vitruvius. On architecture [Granger F, Trans.]. Loeb Classical Library. Cambridge MA: Harvard University Press. vol. 2 Bk. 3 cc. 6, 10, 11.

[14] Nriagu [note 3] pp. 105–16; Needleman & Needleman [note 4] p. 64–94.

[15] Pliny [note 5] Bk XXXIII.31; Nriagu [note 3] pp. 105–16.

[16] Vitruvius [note 14] Bk. VIII. c.3.6; Pliny [note 5] Bk. XXXIV.50; Dioscorides [note 8] Bk. V.9.103.

[17] Nicander. In: Major RH, editor. Classic descriptions of disease. Springfield, IL: CC Thomas; 1959. p. 313. Paul of Aegina. In: Major [note 18] pp. 313.9.

[18] Grandjean [note 12] p. 303–21; Retief & Cilliers [note 2] pp. 167–84.

[19] Scarborough J. The myth of lead poisoning among Romans: an essay reviewed. J Hist Med 1984;39:469–75. Needleman & Needleman [note 4] pp. 64–94.

[20] Gilfillan [note 3] p. 53–60; Needleman & Needleman [note 4] p. 64–94.

[21] Drasch [note 1] pp. 199–231.

RECOMMENDED READING

Drasch GA. Lead burden in prehistorical, historical and modern human bodies. Sci Total Environ 1982;24:199–231.

Emsley J. Ancient world was poisoned by lead. New Sci 1994;142:14.

Gilfillan SC. Lead poisoning and the fall of Rome. J Occup Med 1965;7:53–60.

Grandjean P. Widening perspectives of lead toxicity. Environ Res 1978;17:303–21.

Hodge AT. Vitruvius, lead pipes and lead poisoning. Am J Archaeol 1981;85:486–91.

Needleman L, Needleman D. Lead poisoning and the decline of the Roman aristocracy. Classical Views 1985;29:64–94.

Nicander. Poems and poetical Fragments. [Gow ASF, Scholfield AF, Trans.]. Cambridge: Cambridge University Press; 1953.

Nriagu JD. Occupational exposure to lead in ancient times. Sci Total Environ 1983;32:105–16.

Nriagu JO. Saturnine gout among Roman aristocrats. N Engl J Med 1983;308(11):660–3.

Pliny the Elder. Natural history. [Healy JF, Trans.]. London:Penguin Classics; 1991.

Retief FP, Cilliers L. Loodvergiftiging in antieke Rome. Acta Acad 2000;32(2):167–84.

Scarborough J. The myth of lead poisoning among Romans: an essay reviewed. J Hist Med 1984;39:469–75.

Steinbeck RT. Lead ingestion in ancient times. Palaeopath. Newsletter (Detroit) 1979;27:9–11.

Vitruvius. On Architecture. [Schofield R, Tavernor R, Trans.]. London:Penguin Classics; 2009.

Waldron HA. Lead poisoning in the ancient world. Med Hist 1973;17:391–9.

Waldron T, Wells C. Exposure to lead in the ancient populations. Trans Stud Coll Physicians Phila 1975;1:102–15.

Woolley DE. A perspective of lead poisoning in antiquity and the present. Neurotoxicology 1984;5(3):353–61.

CHAPTER *12*

Poisons, Poisoners, and Poisoning in Ancient Rome

Louise Cilliers and Francois Retief

12.1 SOURCES

Our knowledge of poisonous substances known to the ancient Romans is derived from the records of various contemporary writers. The Greek scholar, Theophrastus, associate and successor of Aristotle as head of the Lyceum (fourth century BC) led the way in identifying plants with medicinal (and poisonous) properties. In the first century AD, Dioscorides of Anazarbus wrote his famous herbal, *De material medica*, which superseded all existing literature in classifying remedies and drugs from the vegetable, animal, and mineral kingdoms. This work, which dealt with close to 1000 drugs, became the standard text for centuries to come. Information on poisons can also be gleaned from the writings of the poet Nicander (second century BC), the army physician Scribonius Largus (1–50 AD), the encyclopedist Pliny the Elder (23–79 AD), another encyclopedist, Cornelius Celsus (first century AD), and the famous physician and philosopher Galen (second century AD) [1].

The Latin word *venenum* is ambiguous and can mean remedy or poison. In fact, in a Roman court jurists demanded that the user of the word *venenum* must add whether it was beneficial or harmful [2]. The ambiguity is due to the fact that the difference between remedy and poison did not necessarily lie in the substance itself but in the dosage. This is clearly illustrated by Dioscorides when he describes the properties and uses of the opium poppy (*Papaver somniferum*), widely employed as a soporific and analgesic; he cautions that if administered in a more concentrated form and greater dosage, it plunges the patient into lethargy and stupor and can even kill. Thus, although in the sixteenth century Paracelsus more formally articulated the principle that the dose makes the poison, it was understood in practice well before his time.

History of Toxicology and Environmental Health. DOI: http://dx.doi.org/10.1016/B978-0-12-800045-8.00013-7

12.2 POISONS

Poisons were of vegetable, animal, or mineral origin [3]. Vegetable poisons were best known and most frequently used. They included plants with belladonna alkaloids such as henbane, thorn apple, deadly nightshade, mandrake, aconite, hemlock, hellebore, yew extract, and opium. It has been suggested that cyanide was in Roman times extracted from the kernels of certain fruits like almonds, but strychnine was unknown to the ancients. The use of figs and mushrooms to dispose of a person was almost certainly based on applying poisons to these foods. If inherently toxic mushrooms had been used, the rapid death of the victim would implicate the *Amonita muscaria* or *Amonita pantherina* kind. Mandragora (mandrake is the common name for this plant genus), with its human-like root, was steeped in superstition: there was a widely shared belief that gathering the root was dangerous, as the plant, when uprooted, uttered a shriek, which caused the death or insanity of those who heard it. However, it was one of the first drugs used effectively as anesthetic and analgesic, rather than as a fatal poison [4]. Hemlock was well known in antiquity, and used as early as the fifth century BC by the law courts of Athens as a legal mode of execution. Socrates died this way in 399 BC. It causes a gradually ascending paralysis and in the end asphyxia when the respiratory organs become paralyzed, and is said to result in an easy and painless death [5]. Aconite was referred to as "the stepmother's poison" or the "mother-in-law's" poison. It was probably used extensively. As little as 3–6 mg is lethal for an adult. It causes rapid onset of symptoms of death due to cardiovascular collapse and respiratory paralysis.

Mineral poisons, for example, salts of lead, mercury, copper, arsenic, and antimony, were known but virtually never used. Fumes from the lead smelting process and from silver and gold mines were recognized as toxic. Poisonous animals were studied by Nicander in his two books on antidotes. The poisons included the venoms of snakes, scorpions, spiders, and insects such as the Spanish fly, as well as such unlikely "poisons" as bull's blood, toads, and salamanders.

The ancients differentiated between three kinds of poisons, namely acute poisons killing rapidly, chronic poisons causing physical deterioration, and chronic poisons causing mental deterioration. Professional poisoners like Locusta, Martina, and Canidia, the infamous trio of women poisoners in Roman times, were often requested by their clients to prepare poisons to suit their specific needs [6]. Poisons were usually administered with food or drink—and for this reason official tasters, *praegustatores* (slaves or freedmen), were employed by the nobility and the wealthy. They became so common that they formed a collegium with a *procurator praegustatorum*. Poisons were also administered by way of enemas, poisoned needles, or a poisoned feather to induce vomiting, as in the case of Emperor Claudius.

12.3 POISONS USED

Pinpointing drugs used in murders (or suicides) recorded in history is difficult, especially when done retrospectively. Descriptions of the mode of death and *post mortem* changes considered typical of poisoning, for example, darkening of the skin and early bloating due to delayed putrefaction, are hardly reliable when related by historians whose sources were at best secondhand. Furthermore, it is likely that combinations of substances were used – it was believed that more substances would be more effective.

In the vast majority of poisonings recorded in ancient Rome, we do not know the nature of the poison or poisons used. However, in the following instances, specific poisons were mentioned [7]:

i. Catuvolcus, the British king mentioned in Caesar's writings, committed suicide by drinking the *sap of the Yew tree.*

ii. The emperor Claudius was killed by poisonous mushrooms or, more probably, *poisoned mushrooms.*

iii. The philosopher Seneca, forced by Nero to commit suicide, took *hemlock* (after unsuccessfully cutting his wrists).

iv. In his novel, *Metamorphoses* (also known as *The Golden Ass*), Apuleius tells of a young man rendered unconscious by *mandragora.*

v. Rumors claim that the emperor, Titus, was poisoned with *sea-hare* (a marine gastropod) by his younger brother Domitian.

vi. Commodus, son of the emperor Marcus Aurelius, killed the Praetorian Prefect, Motilenus, with poisonous figs or *poisoned figs.*

vii. In his satires, Juvenal tells of the woman, Pontia, who boasted among her friends of her ability to kill with *aconite.* Plutarch, on the other hand, tells of one Orodes who was cured of dropsy by taking *aconite.*

12.4 INCIDENTS OF POISONING DURING THE ROMAN REPUBLIC

The following survey of recorded crimes of poisoning reveals the pervasive influence of contemporary sociopolitical circumstances, as well as superstition.

The first recorded incident of poisoning in Rome can be traced back to 331 BC. The city was stricken by a serious pestilence, and rumor had it that the high mortality rate was partly due to poisoning. Though not convinced of the truth of this story, the historian Livy states that a servant girl informed the *curule aedile* that a number of married women conspired to kill a great number of men by means of poison. Twenty prominent women were arrested, but during the trial they stated that they were preparing medications, not poison. When the women were asked to drink these medications themselves, they asked for time to deliberate the request, but soon returned and drank the potion; all died. Eventually, 170 other women were found guilty and executed [8].

During the Second Punic War, the city of Capua revolted against Rome, hoping that Hannibal would come to their aid. It did not happen, and in 211, Capua was taken after a siege. Knowing that they could not expect any mercy, the leader, Virrius, decided to commit suicide, and tried to persuade the senate to do the same. Twenty-seven of the 80 senators complied, and followed Virrius to his home. A meal was prepared during which much wine was imbibed, followed by the poison. They then movingly bade each other farewell and departed to their respective homes. When the Romans entered the city the next morning, the 27 senators had all died. The remaining 53 senators were executed by the Romans [9].

The historian Livy relates the following moving incident: near the end of the Second Punic War the Roman general, Scipio, defeated the Numidian king, Syphax. Syphax's wife, Sophonisba, had in the meantime become involved with Masinissa, one of Scipio's generals. In a desperate attempt to prevent his beloved from being made a Roman captive, Masinissa married Sophonisba. However, just after the ceremony, he was informed that the marriage would not save her. He thus went to his tent and prepared a poisonous potion which he sent to

Sophonisba with the message that his commander had robbed him of the opportunity of fulfilling the first promise that he as bridegroom owed his bride, but that he would stand by his second promise, namely to provide her with the opportunity of evading Roman captivity. She drank the potion and, in a last message to Masinissa, commented on the irony that the same day would commemorate her unconsummated marriage and burial [10].

In 154, two ex-consuls were poisoned by their wives. The senators were becoming uneasy, and assumed jurisdiction over all cases requiring public investigation, such as treason, conspiracy, assassination, and poisoning. At the end of the second century, a court dealing with cases involving poisoning was instituted, and in 80 BC the dictator Sulla promulgated various laws against poisoning. A person would henceforth be guilty if he prepared, sold, or had in his possession dangerous substances [11].

Cicero's speeches provide further evidence of the high incidence of poisoning in his time. In one of the court cases he refers to Oppianicus, who poisoned his wife, brother, and pregnant sister-in-law in order to inherit money; other cases involve Domitius, who murdered his cousin, Fabricius, who wanted to poison a friend, and Catiline, who was guilty of poisoning various people [12].

Pliny tells us that before the battle of Actium (31 BC) Marcus Antonius was so suspicious that he refused any food from Cleopatra unless it was tasted by his personal bodyguard. The queen, however, managed to smuggle a poisoned jug past the bodyguard, but at the last moment, because of her love for Antony, prevented him from drinking it. The cup was then given to a prisoner, who immediately died after drinking it. Plutarch is responsible for the story that Cleopatra committed suicide by the bite of an adder, but it is more likely that she took poison—a snake large enough to kill the queen and two ladies in waiting would have been too large to smuggle past the guards posted there by Octavian to prevent her from committing suicide [13].

This brings us to the end of the Republican era. Four years after the battle of Actium, Octavian became Augustus, the first emperor of the Roman Empire.

12.5 POISONERS AND INCIDENTS OF POISONING DURING THE EMPIRE

12.5.1 Augustus (27 BC—14 AD)

The Julio-Claudian dynasty, which started with Augustus, was infamous for numerous cases of poisoning occurring in the imperial family. Livia, the formidable wife of the emperor, was said by the second century AD historian, Dio Cassius [14], to have poisoned Augustus's grandchildren, Gaius and Lucius Caesar, in order that her own son, Tiberius, would succeed the emperor. There was also a rumor that she had poisoned her aged husband with poisoned figs, but there is no evidence for this [15]. A scandal was exposed when a friend of Augustus, Nonus Asprenas, was arraigned in the senate for the poisoning of 130 guests at a dinner party.

12.5.2 Tiberius (14—37 AD)

In 19 BC, Tiberius's nephew, the popular general Germanicus, died in Asia Minor amid suspicious circumstances, after a quarrel with the governor, Piso, and his wife, Plancina. Germanicus's wife, Agrippina, and his friends stated that he was poisoned by Piso, helped by the infamous poisoner, Martina. The case was referred to the senate in Rome, but on her way to Rome, Martina suddenly died; her body showed no signs of suicide, but during the autopsy, poison was discovered, concealed in a knot in her hair. Poisoning could not be proved during the trial, but Piso was heavily censured and then committed suicide [16].

In 23 AD, Tiberius's son, Drusus, died after a long illness. It was later revealed that he was poisoned by the Praetorian Prefect, Sejanus, who was the lover of the victim's wife, Livilla. Sejanus's wife affirmed under torture that Livilla had prepared a poison which had the effect of physical deterioration over a long period [17]. It is ironic that Germanicus, who probably died a natural death, was believed to have been poisoned, while Drusus, who was poisoned, was believed to have died a natural death.

Sejanus then overreached himself by trying to take over the government while Tiberius was in Capri, but the plot was exposed, and Sejanus and his supporters were all arraigned and executed. Tiberius now became increasingly paranoid and Tacitus relates that many people were accused of treason during mass trials, and committed suicide by poisoning to prevent their families from losing their possessions to the accusers. When the emperor died in Capri, there were rumors that he was poisoned by Gaius (Germanicus's son), but there is little evidence for this [18].

12.5.3 Gaius (Caligula) (37–41 AD)

Dio Cassius tells that this mentally disturbed emperor collected poisons and killed gladiators, jockeys, and horses in his attempt to manipulate these sports in order that his favorites could win [19]. The satirist, Juvenal, claims that his insanity was the result of a love potion administered by his wife, Caesonia [20].

12.5.4 Claudius (41–54 AD)

Claudius probably suffered from congenital cerebral palsy but proved an unexpectedly efficient emperor. Dio Cassius relates that he dumped Gaius's poisons into the sea, which caused the death of scores of fish [21]. It is generally believed that his fourth wife, Agrippina, poisoned him with poisonous or poisoned mushrooms obtained from the poisoner Locusta, to make room for her son, Nero. The 65-year-old ailing emperor did not die immediately, and the physician Xenophon had to use a poisoned feather, ostensibly to make him vomit to get rid of the poison, to finally dispatch him [22].

12.5.5 Nero (54–68 AD)

After the accession of Nero, poisoning among the aristocracy showed a marked increase. The first years of this emotionally unstable young emperor's reign, when the philosopher Seneca was his counselor, were irreproachable, but Seneca's influence started waning as Nero grew up. Seneca was eventually unfairly accused of conspiracy and forced to commit suicide by poison; after opening his arteries he took hemlock which also did not have the desired immediate effect and he was thus smothered in a steam bath [23]. The later years of Nero's principate, when he was under the influence of the evil Tigellinus, Prefect of the Praetorian Guard, became an orgy of murders. The historians Suetonius [24], Tacitus [25], and Dio Cassius [26] tell of the deaths (by poison) of Nero's stepbrother, Britannicus; Silanus, governor of Asia; Domitia, his aunt whose riches he desired; Burrus, Prefect of the Praetorian Guard; and Pallas and other freedmen. Nero also got rid of his meddlesome mother, Agrippina, but could not use poison since she had for some time been using antidotes to make her immune; he thus had her brutally beaten to death after she had swum to shore when the planned shipwreck which was to have disposed of her went awry [27].

Nero's poisons were usually prepared by Locusta. Her death penalty was suspended after the murder of Britannicus and various others, and she was appointed the emperor's adviser on poisons, and allowed to establish a school of poisoning where she could train others in her art. Locusta tested her poisons on animals and convicted criminals [28].

12.5.6 The Flavian Dynasty (69–96 AD)

According to historians the number of poisonings decreased after Nero's death, but there were still some incidents during the next two centuries which will be dealt with. After Nero came the notorious Year of the Four Emperors (69) with armies from all over the empire trying to raise their generals to the throne. Then followed the Flavian dynasty, of which the cruel, unstable younger son, *Domitian*, became emperor in 81 AD. He was accused of poisoning his elder brother, the emperor *Titus* (who died unexpectedly at the age of 42), with sea-hare (a marine gastropod). It is, however, more likely that Titus died of malaria while besieging Jerusalem [29]. Another suspicious death was that of Agricola, the popular Roman governor in Britain, who died in 93 amid suspicious circumstances. It was well known that Domitian was jealous of him, and when physicians from Rome visited Agricola during his last illness, the rumor originated that the emperor had arranged that he be poisoned. However, Tacitus could find no conclusive evidence [30].

12.5.7 Hadrian (117–138 AD)

This capable emperor had an unhappy married life, probably because of his homosexual inclination. When his wife, Sabina, died in 136 AD, it was widely believed that he had poisoned her. At a later stage when the emperor himself suffered from serious edema, he tried to commit suicide but the weapon was taken from him; he then asked his physician to provide poison, but rather than accede to the request, the physician killed himself [31].

12.5.8 Commodus (180–192 AD)

Unlike his father, Marcus Aurelius, Commodus was a failure as emperor. It is said that he poisoned the Prefect of the Praetorian Guard, Motilenus, with poisoned figs. Eventually, during a conspiracy,

Commodus's favorite concubine, Marcia, tried to poison him, but the poison only made him drowsy, and thereafter he began vomiting. When it became evident that he was not going to die, he was strangled by the athlete Narcissus [32].

12.5.9 Caracalla (211−217 AD)

Caracalla's reign began with the murder of his brother, Geta, who was designated co-emperor in the will of their father, Septimius Severus. Geta was popular and had many supporters, who were mercilessly dispatched after his death, mostly by sword, but also by poisoning. It was said that 20,000 people died during Caracalla's reign [33].

12.6 CONCLUSION

The survey of recorded crimes by poison underlines the pervasive influence of contemporary sociopolitical circumstances [34]. Incidents of poisoning in early Rome usually coincided with crises such as wars and epidemics; superstition and the belief that scapegoats would solve the problem would have been determining factors. This phase was gradually superseded by a very well-documented era in which countless individual cases of poisoning are reported, and which reached a peak during the reign of the Julio-Claudian emperors in the first century AD. Apart from the influence of personal factors such as paranoid and mentally unstable emperors, the transition from Republic to Empire was a politically unstable period which created much tension, and thwarted ambition led to numerous political intrigues and murders. During the reign of the so-called Five Good Emperors in the second century AD, commonly regarded as the most prosperous period in Roman history, there was a significant decline in poisoning and suicides by poison. Granted that this period is less well documented, the political stability of this era, which would have brought a greater degree of peace of mind, could have been a determining factor in the decline of violent deaths.

REFERENCES

[1] Hornblower S, Spawforth A. The Oxford classical dictionary. 3rd ed. Oxford: Oxford University Press; 1996.

[2] Kaufman DB. Poisons and poisoning among the Romans. Class Philol 1932;27:156. Horstmanshoff HFJ. Ancient medicine between hope and fear: medicament, magic and poison in the Roman Empire. Eur Rev 1999;7(1):43.

[3] Cilliers L, Retief FPR. Poisons, poisoning and the drug trade in ancient Rome. Akroterion 2000;45:91−5.

[4] Cilliers L. Anaesthesia and analgesia in ancient Greece and Rome (c. 400 BCE−300 CE). In: Askitopoulou H, editor. Proceedings of the seventh international symposium on the history of anaesthesia. Heraklion: Crete University Press; 2012. pp. 31−44.

[5] Cilliers [note 4] pp. 31−44.

[6] Cilliers and Retief [note 3] p. 90.

[7] For more details see Cilliers and Retief [note 3] pp. 96−7.

[8] Livy. History of Rome. [Foster BO, Trans.]. Loeb Classical Library, vol. IV. Cambridge, MA: Harvard University Press; 1926, Bk.8 c.18.

[9] Livy [note 8] Bk. 26 cc. 13−14.

[10] Livy [note 8] Bk. 30 cc. 12−15.

[11] Scullard HH. From the Gracchi to Nero: a history of Rome from 133 BC to AD 68. London: Methuen; 1982. p. 86.

[12] Cicero. Orations. Pro Cluentio et al., In Catilinam I-IV, Philippics [Hodge HG, Kerr WCA, Trans.]. Loeb Classical Library, vols. IX, X, and XV. Cambridge, MA: Harvard University Press.

[13] Plutarch. Antony [Perrin B, Trans.] Loeb Classical Library, vol. IX. Cambridge, MA: Harvard University Press; 1920, c.86. Retief FP, Cilliers L. Dood van Kleopatra [Death of Cleopatra]. Geneeskunde 1999;4(1): 8−11.

[14] Roman history [Cary E, Trans.]. Loeb Classical Library, vol. VII. Cambridge, MA: Harvard University Press; 1924, Bk. 56 c. 30.2.

[15] Tacitus. Annals [Moore Ch, Trans.]. Loeb Classical Library, vol. III. Cambridge, MA: Harvard University Press; 1931, Bk. 1, cc. 5.1−3.

[16] Tacitus Annals [note 15] Bk. III. cc. 7.12−15.

[17] Tacitus Annals [note 15] Bk. IV. c. 8.

[18] Suetonius Tiberius [Bradley KR, Trans.]. Loeb Classical Library, vol. I. Cambridge, MA: Harvard University Press; 1998, c.73.

[19] Roman History [note 14] Bk LIX c.14.

[20] Satires [Braund SM, Trans.]. Loeb Classical Library. Cambridge, MA: Harvard University Press. 2004, Sat. VI. Lines 610−626.

[21] Roman History [note 14] Bk LIX 14.

[22] Tacitus Annals [note 15] Bk. XII. cc. 66−67.

[23] Tacitus Annals [note 15] Bk. XV cc. 60−62.

[24] Nero [note 18] c. 35.5.

[25] Annals [note 15] Bk. XIII.c.1.

[26] Roman history [note 14] Bk LXI c.7.4.

[27] Tacitus Annals [note 15] Bk. XIV cc. 7−8.

[28] Suetonius, Claudius [Bradley KR, Trans.]. Loeb Classical Library, vol. II. Cambridge, MA: Harvard University Press. 1998, c.44. Ibid. Nero c.33.3.

[29] Thompson CJS. Poisons and poisoning. New York, NY: Macmillan & Co.; 1931. pp. 67−8.

[30] Tacitus Agricola [Ogilvie RM, et al., Trans.]. Loeb Classical Library, vol. I. Cambridge, MA: Harvard University Press; 1970, c.43.

[31] Spartianus. Augustan history. Lives of the Later Caesars [Birley A, Trans.]. Penguin Classics, 1976, cc. 23–26.

[32] Lampridius. Commodus. In: Chronicle of the Roman Empire [Scarre C, Trans.]. London: Thames & Hudson. 1995, c.9.

[33] Lampridius. Caracalla [note 32] c.3.

[34] Cilliers and Retief [note 3] pp. 98–9.

Printed and bound by CPI Group (UK) Ltd, Croydon, CR0 4YY

03/10/2024

01040423-0016